How to Find Relief from

Migraine

How to Find Relief from

Migraine

by

ROSEMARY DUDLEY
and Wade Rowland

A Nicholson Press Book

COLLINS
Toronto

First Published in 1981 by
Wm. Collins Sons & Co. Canada Ltd.
100 Lesmill Road
Don Mills, Ontario
Canada M3B 2T5

Canadian Cataloguing in Publication Data

Dudley, Rosemary.
   How to find relief from migraine

ISBN 0-00216819-7

1. Migraine.   2. Migraine—Prevention.
3. Migraine—Homeopathic treatment.
I. Rowland, Wade, 1944-   II. Title.

RC392.D82   616.8'57   C81-094764-1

The Nicholson Press
9 Sultan Street
Toronto, Ontario M5S 1L6

Editor: Conrad Wieczorek
Designer: Keith Abraham

Printed in the United States of America

TABLE OF CONTENTS

INTRODUCTION

In an article published in the journal *Headache*† Dr. Russell Packard, a psychiatrist, asked and answered the question "What Does the Headache Patient Want?" He found, perhaps surprisingly, that pain relief was not at the top of most headache patients' agenda. Rather, most headache sufferers wanted an explanation of what their headaches were and why they were occurring, together with reassurance that they did not have an ominous lesion such as a brain tumor. Treatment was accorded second place in these peoples' expectations.

To what extent do the health care professions, notably medicine, meet these expectations?

There is little doubt that in nearly all cases physicians do effectively reassure people that they do not have as causes for their headaches serious conditions such as brain tumors, aneurysms, meningitis, or other diseases. Most physicians have enough training and experience that by carefully questioning their patients they can elicit enough facts about the headache to allow the diagnosis to begin to take shape. (Patients, incidentally, should realize that it is this history-taking that is the crucial part of the diagnostic process. The physician depends on information given by the patient. If the patient's description is vague and inexact—in medical parlance "an exodontal history"; that is, like pulling teeth to get any useful information—then the diagnosis is

†The Journal of the American Association For The Study Of Headache—Ref. *Headache* Vol. 19:370, 1979.

likely to be equally vague and inexact). The diagnosis is then confirmed by a careful physical examination and, if necessary, by selected neurological investigations such as skull x-rays and brain scans. This diagnostic process will establish, in well over 95% of patients, that the headaches are not due to serious disease but rather to the malfunctioning of structurally normal tissues. Examples of such malfunction are the dilation and stretching of scalp blood vessels that may culminate in migraine, and the sustained contraction of muscles of the scalp and neck that can lead to tension headache. Physicians are usually reasonably effective also in relieving most peoples' headache pain. This may not seem so to many of the readers of this book, but most people who buy and read this book will do so primarily because their headaches are still a problem to them. The fact remains that well over three-quarters of all patients with head-aches can expect substantial relief of their symptom from appropriate application by competent health care professionals of medication and other therapeutic modalities now available. This figure improves all the time as new drugs, new techniques and new procedures are developed, and as more and more physicians become more and more expert in the diagnosis and treatment of headache through attendance at postgraduate courses and the reading of headache journals.

Where the health professions fall short of the mark is in educating their patients about exactly what their headaches are, what may be bringing them on, and what the patient can do to minimize the frequency and severity of symptoms. With complete truth the professionals plead lack of time. There are simply not enough hours in the day to sit down with every patient with headaches and explain in detail everything that the patient wants to know. Nor is it a good idea that the patient regard the physician as the sole source of information and help. This can foster a dependency situation in which patients, by calling on the doctor for each and every headache, or by questioning him about the subtlest detail ("should I go to cousin Susan's wedding next week?—I might get a headache") abdicate responsibility for their own lives and become passive recipients of care rather than active partners in treatment.

Rosemary Dudley encountered this information gap many years ago, and has since devoted a good portion of her adult life to filling it in. She is admirably qualified to do so. Not only is she herself a migraine sufferer, with first-hand knowledge of the pain and frustration that is the lot of the patient with headache, but she is an expert in communication—she has served as information officer to highly placed government figures, and has been successful in the demanding field of public relations.

Her major contribution to the fight against headache has been the establishment of The Migraine Foundation. In the few years since its beginning, The Migraine Foundation has given to many thousands of migraine sufferers detailed information, not only by brochure but by personal telephone conversation, about migraine and other kinds of headaches, why they occur, and what the patient can do about them. Possibly even more importantly, the Foundation has initiated with the media numerous television and radio presentations, and newspaper and magazine articles, about headaches, their causes and consequences, and about the plight of the headache sufferer. This coverage, within a short period of time, has transformed the image of the migraine sufferer from one of a manipulative and self-indulgent neurotic to one of a person with a genuine medical disorder frequently susceptible to treatment. None of this would have happened without Miss Dudley's enthusiasm, determination and evangelical spirit.

This book is an extension of Rosemary's drive to inform the public in general, and migraine sufferers in particular, about headache. It deals with the magnitude of the problem that migraine poses to society and to the individual; the many causes of headache; and most significantly, how the patient, working with health professionals, can reduce the toll that migraine takes. It gives the migraine sufferer information that will help him or her cope better with the many aspects of migraine.

John Edmeads, M.D., F.R.C.P. (C)., F.A.C.P.

AUTHOR'S PREFACE

"The tests are all negative."

This called for an expelling of the breath you'd been holding in...for weeks, it seemed. A raw, cold, rainy and overcast February had brought with it what had verged on being a continuous four-week headache. You had had headaches before, many, many headaches, but never one so prolonged and severe.

It still took a few minutes before it sunk in that there was *no* brain tumour; that neither death nor invalidism (the horrific idea of the decline into a vegetative state that had stalked the 2 a.m. imagination) was to be found in the prognosis.

The best reply you could muster was, "Oh."

The word "migraine" was dimly heard. Your mind created a scene for a Victorian novel, the heroine reclining, Camille-like, on chaise longue, a cloth dipped in vinegar held to the perfectly-coiffed head..."Madame is not receiving today," she informs the staff.

After three weeks in hospital and all those tests, migraine was not the kind of diagnosis you had expected to come away with.

You ought to have been jumping for joy (the pain in the head permitting). You ought to have been effusive in the gratitude you felt; the appreciation for all that had been done for you by the patient hospital staff.

It is months later before you can define your thoughts clearly. The first clue should have been obvious: contrary to your ideas of hospitals as places of healing (you had come home cured after an emergency appendix attack at age ten), this time you had been discharged with a shiny new diagnosis, but with the head pain still present. But then you had three prescriptions, and surely these were going to do wonders.

Later the original prescriptions had been exchanged for different medications. But still the attacks continued, interfering more and more with day-to-day living.

You realized now that the diagnosis amounted to a lifetime sentence with no time off for good behaviour . . . nothing but the suggestion that, "after menopause, you might find that the attacks ease." Menopause! But you are not yet thirty!

And one day, with tears of pain and frustration streaming, you say it aloud: Why couldn't they have found something wrong . . . something they could have fixed, patched up, repaired, operated on? A nice, gentle, benign tumour . . . even if it meant sacrificing some minor motor function. Why did it have to be "only migraine?" And the idea makes you feel terribly guilty and unworthy.

And one day, you find yourself saying, "God, take me now," and you cannot believe it is your own voice, not this first time. You were supposed to be Bette Davis in *Dark Victory,* able to face even certain death with every hair in place and a smile playing on the lips. Suffering was supposed to be glamorous. But you are discovering that there is no glamour involved in having migraine, in upchucking expensive steak and wine all over somebody else's shoes; in staying home with the curtains drawn, phone off the hook, wondering how you are going to make it to work the following day.

You think, "When this one has passed. . . ." And it will pass, won't it? They have always passed before. Yes, it will pass. But what if it does not? What did Dorothy Parker say about suicide? "Guns aren't lawful;/ Nooses give;/ Gas smells awful;/ You might as well live." Did it ever hurt Dorothy Parker just to *think*?

And the thing is that apart from this *condition,* you are healthy, able to go without sleep, eager to dance nights away, quick to pack suitcases and tear off to meetings, conventions, conferences where exciting plans are being made for the future of the post-war nation . . . .

The early signs of migraine had gone unrecognized: the occasional unexplained tummy ache, the queasy feeling that sometimes came with eating certain foods, or leaving sunglasses behind; that once-a-month headache which was "part of being a woman," they said. As a teenager, working Saturdays, you'd spent at least half your money on those little snap-up boxes of aspirin, but they were advertised everywhere and everyone carried them, just like the clean handkerchief there in your purse . . . .

But now you know, it is migraine. And, eventually, you realize you do not even know what migraine really is, so you begin to try to find out.

Looking back over the past twenty years, I realize that I was fortunate. Physicians who *cared* never gave up on me, never ceased trying various medications and therapies. And one day I answered a call for migraine sufferers to volunteer for a research project. I felt I had nothing to lose, and perhaps a lot to gain. Some two hundred sufferers were duly interviewed, and ten were selected for initial hospitalization. The tests were being done in a world-renowned institution devoted to the care of children, and this led to some amusing vignettes: my five-foot-two frame on a four-foot trolly, being transported on a hospital elevator during visiting hours. As I was being wheeled off, I could think of nothing to say to the astonished parents but: "I matured late in life."

Because of the lab reports on my blood and other testing (for which I can take no credit) I was invited to become *the* volunteer, which meant checking into the hospital each time a migraine began. I got the same room each time, the muted blue walls decorated with Little Bo-Peep cut-outs.

This was a turning point. During the hours and days when I was asked to go without medication, the researchers kindly directed my thoughts away from the pain with talk about the state of migraine research around the world, and by describing the fledgling international network of neurologists interested in migraine. For me, it was like Christmas morning, to find out that so much work had been done and that so much more was waiting only for financing and personnel (and, to a degree, for increased interest, especially from the public.) In those discussions lay the beginnings of the Migraine Foundation.

What follows in the pages to come is a distillation of the knowledge gained from my subsequent interest and involvement. During the past decade we have been in contact with over 280,000 migraine sufferers through letters, the telephone, lectures, media appearances and so on. Their comments, complaints, histories and suggestions provide a deep well of personal experience on which we have been able to draw in preparing this manuscript. Other material has been gleaned from the growing volume of research material being turned out by the worldwide medical profession.

I am deeply indebted to the support and guidance of the Migraine Foundation's Board of Directors (who without outward flinching have allowed our service to sufferers to outgrow our resources, thus creating an initial, rather large, deficit). And to those physicians serving on our Medical Advisory Committee: they have been both patient and generous in undertaking the education of this lay person.

Although this book has been written on Migraine Foundation time, and proceeds from its publication will be devoted to migraine work, none of the physicians associated with the Foundation should be held responsible in any way for the comments found herein. Such as they are, they are mine, and are presented by me as a migraine sufferer, with the sole purpose of discussing migraine with other sufferers.

I'm very glad, today, that The Almighty did not "take me now," but instead allowed me to play a small part in increasing public understanding of headache, and what it can mean to those who suffer.

Rosemary Dudley,
Toronto

CHAPTER 1

An Introduction to Migraine

Now, friends, if you want to try something really unusual, try passing out in front of five thousand people. Fortunately, the boys in my band have learned to tell when it's coming. They just take me by the elbow and help me sit until it passes, or else they help me off the stage. One time I was off the stage about forty-five minutes, and when I came back, Don Ballinger and the boys had done such a good job playing and joking that nobody cared whether I came back or not.

But what bothered me was hearing some fans afterward. "She must have been drunk," some fans said. . . . Can you believe it? They thought I was drunk. Now when I don't feel good I make an announcement that I've got a migraine, but there're people who still don't believe it.

Loretta Lynn, *Coal Miner's Daughter*

A neurologist once observed of migraine: "Perhaps no other condition so disrupts the lives of its victims and yet evokes so little sympathy and compassion for the afflicted. Few other victims of legitimate disease are subjected to as much skepticism regarding their symptoms."

It's difficult for loved ones, employers, workmates and friends of the migraine sufferer to identify with someone who is incapacitated by what they perceive to be a mere headache. Unless, that is, they have experienced a migraine attack themselves. There is no obvious or easily understandable cause—no virus going around, no physical injury, and beyond the obvious distress of the sufferer, there are seldom any symptoms that can be easily observed by the uninformed outsider. There is no wound, no bleeding, no blisters or rash. The attacks come and go, leaving the victim apparently healthy between bouts. As far as anyone can see, it is just a bad headache, and what most people do when they have a bad headache is to take a couple of aspirin and try to ignore it until it goes away.

However, this procedure seldom solves anything for the migraine sufferer, and the unfortunate conclusion often arrived at by the uninformed bystander is that the victim is somehow deriving a perverse, neurotic enjoyment from the pain, perhaps that he is permitting the pain to continue in order to punish those around him, by disrupting their lives. "Not tonight dear, I've got a splitting headache," is a common complaint; for those who don't understand, it comes across as game playing, as an excuse instead of a valid reason. More seriously, the sensitive partner or spouse may conclude that he or she is responsible for the pain, especially if the sufferer is unable to point to any other obvious cause.

The result of the widespread ignorance of the causes and effects of migraine has been that millions of sufferers the world over are compelled to lead lives of quiet despair, burdened with pain that they themselves do not fully understand and that those around them comprehend even less. Guilt, depression and anger can become constant companions both for the sufferer and for those close to him or her. Withdrawal and loneliness can grow to dangerous dimensions; for those who are married, separation and divorce are not uncommon spin-offs of migraine.

Most of this toll in suffering can be avoided, and we feel certain that it will be avoided in future simply through better public understanding of what migraine is all about.

It's difficult to believe that so much ignorance continues to surround a condition that is at least as old as recorded history and which today, by conservative estimate, affects 20% of the world's population; nevertheless, that's the way it really is.

Migraine has been accurately described in some of the oldest writings known to archaeology. More than five thousand years ago, a Sumerian scribe recorded on a clay tablet the following lines:

Headache roameth over the desert; blowing like the wind,
Flashing like lightning, it is loosed above and below;
It cutteth off him who feareth not his god; like a reed,
Like a stalk of henna it slitteth his sinews.
It wasteth the flesh of him who hath no protecting goddess;
Flashing like a heavenly star, it cometh like the dew;
It standeth hostile against the wayfarer, scorching him like
 the day.
This man it hath struck, and
Like one with heart disease, he staggereth;
Like one bereft of reason he is broken;
Like one which has been cast into the fire he is shrivelled;
Like a wild ass . . . his eyes are full of cloud;
On himself he feedeth, bound in death;
Headache whose course, like the dread windstorm, none
 knoweth,
None knoweth its full time or bond.

And there is this Sumerian priest-physician's formula for relief, also more than five thousand years old:

Take the hair of a virgin kid;
Let a wise woman spin it on the right side
And double it on the left;
Bind twice seven knots.
Then perform the incantation of Eridu;
Bind therewith the head of the sick man;
Bind therewith his life.
Cast the water of the incantation over him,
That the headache may ascend to heaven.

A more dramatic treatment has been utilized down through the centuries in the form of trepanning—the drilling of a small hole in the vault of the skull, presumably to release the evil spirit responsible for the pain. Skulls showing evidence of trepanning and dating back to the late Stone Age have been found in Asia, in Europe and in North and South America. In Melanesia in the South Pacific, trepanning persisted until modern times as a treatment for insanity, epilepsy and chronic headache.

With Hippocrates (460-357 BC) and the beginnings of the scientific era of medicine came this description of a headache, almost certainly migrainous:

Most of the time he seemed to see something shining before him like a light, usually in part of the right eye; at the end of a moment, a violent pain supervened in the right temple, then in all the head and neck, where the head is attached to the spine . . . vomiting, when it became possible, was able to divert the pain and render it moderate.

By the beginning of the second century AD, Aretaeus, a physician practising in Alexandria, had described migraine vividly and precisely, noting that, "It is an illness by no means mild, even though it intermits, and though it appears to be slight." Shortly thereafter Galen (AD 131-200) gave the one-sided headache the name *hemicrania*; from this came the Old English *megrim* and the French *migraine*, which is now in common use.

But despite the condition's ancient lineage, a modern specialist was moved to say recently—and ruefully—that, "Ten years ago we knew enough about migraine to fill the back of a postcard. Today, we know enough to fill the back of two post-cards." His frustration accurately reflects that of many migraine victims who have been unable to find relief.

There is an anecdote told of George Bernard Shaw, with which sufferers will be able to identify. About once a month, until he was seventy, Shaw suffered a devastating headache which lasted for a whole day. It was while he was recovering from one of these bouts that he was first introduced to George Nansen, the famous Arctic explorer. Shaw asked him if he had ever discovered a cure for headache. Nansen, amazed, could only reply: "No, I haven't." "Have you ever *tried* to find a cure for headache?" Again, Nansen could only report that he hadn't. "Well," Shaw exploded, "that is the most amazing thing! You have spent your life in trying to discover the North Pole, which nobody on earth cares tuppence about, and you have never attempted to discover a cure for the headache, which every living person is crying aloud for." Unfortunately, Nansen's response is not recorded.

Although it remains true that there is no cure for migraine, modern investigation of the condition has progressed to the point where it is now possible to offer substantial relief to most migraine sufferers. And, perhaps as important, enough is now known about the characteristics of migraine and its frequency in the population that the sufferer need no longer bear the additional psychological burdens so often associated with the affliction.

Some pertinent facts about migraine:
- About one in four people have experienced a migraine attack. You are not alone.
- Migraine is, for the most part, an inherited disorder of the vascular system: it is a physical disease. It is not a psychosomatic or neurotic condition (although external stresses can sometimes trigger an attack).
- About 15% of all migraine attacks are suffered by children and adolescents fifteen years of age and under. Sadly enough, even infants are sometimes victims. But symptoms most often become acute between the ages of twenty-seven and thirty-five.
- Migraine headaches hurt more than other headaches— a great deal more. This is because the body's internal pain regulating mechanism is disrupted by chemical changes that take place in the body during an attack.
- There is no such thing as the "migraine personality." Migraine sufferers are neither more nor less intelligent, compulsive, hard-working, talented, dour, depressive, introverted, silly or

wise than the rest of the population. Surveys which have purported to demonstrate otherwise have been shown conclusively to have been inaccurate, for a variety of reasons. In fact, it is difficult to see how this particular myth has persisted, given the diversity of personality types represented in even a brief list of some of the more famous sufferers of migraine: Thomas Jefferson, Ulysses S. Grant, Frederic Chopin, Charles Darwin, Sigmund Freud, Virginia Woolf, David Frost. In most cases, the only thing these men and women have in common with each other is their illness.

• The symptoms of migraine can be dramatic and frightening. They can mimic the symptoms of life-threatening diseases such as brain tumor and stroke. Temporary paralysis and partial or even complete short-term loss of vision are uncommon, though not-unheard-of accompaniments. But migraine almost never causes permanent disability, and sufferers are generally perfectly healthy between attacks. Doctors report that of *all* patients with headache, less than 3% have their headaches on the basis of ominous disease.

• Although most often experienced as head pain, migraine can also cause severe pain in the abdomen and, in adolescent boys (and some girls), sharp leg pain following strenuous exercise.

• Although more women than men suffer from migraine, the preponderance is not nearly so great as was once thought. And the difference that does exist is probably almost entirely attributable to the fact that, in women, migraine can be triggered by hormonal upsets such as those which occur during menstruation, ovulation, menopause and from taking birth control pills. What is clear is that men are far more prone than women to try to ignore or conceal their migraines, and less likely to seek medical help. They therefore tend to be statistically under-reported.

• One final relevant fact: It is now possible for most migraine sufferers to reduce the frequency and severity of their attacks, possibly by half, either through self-help, or through self-help assisted by medication. Not infrequently, the attacks can be eliminated almost completely.

The first and sometimes the most difficult step in the process is to obtain a valid diagnosis from a physician. Because the symptoms of migraine are observable only during an attack, the physician must rely on information provided by the patient. The rule when visiting a doctor is: "Have your symptoms ready."

If medication is needed, it is important to persist until you and your physician find the drug that works for you. Migraine is a highly individualistic condition; what works for one person may have no effect at all on another. Finding the correct medication and dosage may take time.

In many cases, migraine attacks can be reduced in severity and frequency, or even eliminated, through the avoidance of migraine "triggers." There are many such triggers, ranging from foods like chocolate, cheeses, citrus fruits and smoked meats, to abrupt changes in barometric pressure, to bright lights, noise and stress. Not all of these affect every migraine sufferer. What is important is to isolate those which affect you and to learn to avoid them.

CHAPTER 2

Why me? Who gets Migraine, and Why

First come shimmering blind spots in my field of vision, which bring with them immediately the horrible realization that this might be the beginning of a twenty-four-hour period of suffering, when all activities come to a standstill. There are still some minutes of grace which can be used for getting out of heavy traffic, for cancelling an appointment, or informing my wife of the impending calamity. Not much time remains: soon the blind spots develop into turning cogwheels, jagged lines and bright flashes. Sometimes objects are elongated or compressed out of all recognition, as in a surrealist painting. I sometimes have difficulty speaking intelligibly, or understanding the speech of others. There is still some faint hope that all this might end abortively, without developing into a full-scale attack. But then the pain begins, with a severe, generalized or one-sided headache which is increased by any movement of the head. It is accompanied by coldness to the point of goose flesh and shivering, lasting three to four minutes, alternating with sweating—especially on the face and neck—for the same duration. I am restless and feel indescribably wretched and ill. After about twenty minutes of these initial symptoms, waves of nausea begin. The effort of getting rapidly to the bathroom makes the headache and other symptoms still worse, as do the strains of vomiting and retching. I stumble back to the bed, shivering, pale and haggard and literally willing to die. For the next two or three hours, this dismal process is repeated every quarter hour or so, any consecutive thought or mental activity is out of the question, and sensitivity to light and noise is extreme. Gradually the intervals between retching lengthen, and snatches of sleep become possible. By the afternoon, the head pain has improved, and the hot and cold flashes have ceased. But the nausea remains, as does the mental lethargy and confusion. By early evening there is a decided improvement, and the headache is gone. When I get out of bed I am still shaky and uncoordinated, and mentally vague and sluggish. . . quite incapable of sustained conversation or even of answering the telephone. I am also thirsty; however, the smell of food is almost intolerable. All I really want is more sleep. It may take another full day for the symptoms to disappear completely.†

Almost everybody gets a headache now and then. The kind of headache most people get most often is the so-called tension headache—really a muscle-contraction headache. The pain results from the sustained contraction of the muscles of the scalp, face, jaw and neck, and it is likely to be moderate in intensity, but prolonged. Most people are susceptible when they are harassed or mentally fatigued, although the headaches can also come from a variety of physical circumstances such as long hours of uncomfortable confinement in an airplane or automobile. Almost everyone knows how to treat these headaches: eliminate the stress or physical discomfort if possible; perhaps take some over-the-counter analgesic; apply heat and massage to the back of the neck and shoulders. To the extent that it promotes relaxation, alcohol in moderation can sometimes help,

---

†A doctor describes his own migraine attacks. Adapted from *Sick Doctors*. (Heinemann Heath, Raymond Greene, ed., London, 1971). By permission of the publishers.

too. If none of this brings relief, the possibility of migraine should be investigated.

Many people get headaches which they describe as "sinus headaches," and they treat them with various nationally-advertised patent medicines which claim to offer relief. But the majority of people who think they have sinus headaches really have either a form of muscle contraction headache, migraine, or allergy-related headache. True sinus headache is quite rare, and where it is present, an X-ray will usually reveal that a blockage has occurred. The affected sinus may then have to be drained by means of a minor surgical procedure.

Headache may also result from a variety of serious medical conditions, such as severe hypertension or high blood pressure, anemia, meningitis (an inflammation of the inner lining of the skull), brain hemorrhage, impending stroke, glaucoma and serious dental problems. But doctors report that less than 3% of patients complaining of headache are suffering from any of these ominous conditions.

However, the symptoms of many of the dangerous medical problems associated with head pain may often closely mimic migraine and vice versa. This provides the best possible reason for having your headache problem properly diagnosed by a competent physician. Self-diagnosis is always risky.

At one time the diagnosis of migraine was done almost entirely by exclusion: that is, tests were conducted to check for a whole range of serious diseases associated with head pain, and if none was found, it was concluded that the headache might be migrainous. Today, with a deeper and more widespread understanding of migraine and its symptoms, doctors are usually able to diagnose the condition directly, without recourse to large numbers of tedious, expensive and occasionally painful tests, especially if the head pain has persisted for some time. However, the role played by the patient in such a diagnosis is very important: he or she must be prepared to provide the doctor with a detailed description of the headaches—their location, frequency, duration and intensity and any suspected causes or triggers. It is also important for the patient to find out whether or not there is a family history of headache: this is often the single most important clue to the diagnosis of migraine.

CLASSIC MIGRAINE

There are two distinct stages to a classic migraine attack: the *pre-headache* or *prodrome* stage (prodrome meaning going before) and the headache itself. Symptoms vary widely with the individual, but, in general, the pre-headache stage—called the *aura*—is characterized by unusual visual phenomena. These may range all the way from a slightly increased sensitivity to bright light, to blank spots in the field of vision, to dramatic and disorienting distortions of size and shape. People or objects or parts of the sufferer's own body may appear to grow smaller or larger in *Alice in Wonderland* style. Lewis Carroll was a migraine sufferer, and it is suspected that his prodrome experiences may have provided the basis for some of Alice's adventures. Many who have experienced a classic migraine attack are struck by the similarity between their own visual experiences and the original John Tenniel illustrations for *Alice,* which were done under Carroll's direct supervision.

But most commonly the visual effects—called the *scotoma*—consist of brightly flashing or glittering lights which may resolve themselves into shimmering zigzag patterns across the field of vision. Ragged blind spots may cause words to vanish from printed pages and furniture and other obstructions to disappear as they are approached.

Some report a feeling of numbness or weakness on one side of the body during the pre-headache stage; others, a general clumsiness and lack of co-ordination which may resemble the effects of drunkenness. There are victims who find themselves unable to remember words, or to form coherent sentences. Some people become energetic; others lethargic and drowsy, yawning frequently. Some feel elated to the point of euphoria; others are overcome by depression and irritability. Often, just before the onset of the headache, the hands and feet become puffy and cold.

The pre-headache phase can last anywhere from five minutes to an hour, and sometimes the visual phenomena, speech impairment and other disabilities disappear with the arrival of the headache. But this is not always the case: there may be some overlapping.

The headache itself is usually, but not always, one-sided. In its early stages it is commonly marked by a throbbing which becomes worse with each beat of the pulse. This may later change to a constant pain. This pain may settle around the forehead, or the top of the head, or behind, over, or in one or both eyes or temples. Occasionally it will affect the face below the eye, spreading to the cheek, nostril, ear, jaw and even gums. The pain can range from mild to very severe. It can last anywhere from a few hours to several days and is sometimes accompanied by nausea. Some report that vomiting temporarily eases the pain, or that it may even eliminate it. Often there is a flu-like achiness throughout the body, and chills and the sensation of feverishness are common, as are cold hands and feet. Constipation and diarrhea are both common in the early stages of the headache. The hands, feet and abdomen may swell with retained body fluids so that shoes no longer fit, and belts begin to pinch. The face may become puffy and the eyes bloodshot. Pallor is usual. Most sufferers experience an intense aversion to light and noise and crave nothing so much as a quiet, darkened room with a place to lie down and a pillow to keep the head elevated. Many also develop a similarly intense aversion to strong odors, particularly those of food. The blood vessels may stand out prominently, and the face, neck and scalp are often tender to the touch.

A recent study in Florence, Italy has confirmed what many sufferers know but seldom talk about—even to their doctors. And that is that a significant proportion of migraine sufferers experience intense sexual arousal as one of the body's chemical reactions during an attack. It may occur at the beginning of the process but happens more often toward the end, especially if the attack has lasted for days.

As the headache begins to ease, there may be increased urination as the body rids itself of fluids retained earlier in the attack. The hangover or washed-out feeling that generally follows an attack can last a day or more: on the other hand, some sufferers enjoy euphoria and a sense of well-being following an attack.

Depending on the individual, another attack may occur within hours or days—or it may be weeks, months, even years before the next one comes along. (Migraine attacks are more frequently reported in the spring and fall than at other times of the year.) Between attacks, most sufferers enjoy ordinary good health. Permanent debilitation due to migraine is extremely rare; but it should be underlined that a prolonged, severe migraine attack can be considered a medical emergency sometimes requiring hospitalization so that the victim can be carefully watched and so that potent pain killers can be administered under direct medical supervision.

COMMON MIGRAINE

Because of the involvement of all the senses, especially vision, classic migraine is frequently described in detail although only 15% of sufferers experience this type of migraine. The rest, diagnosed as having "common" migraine, generally find that the first obvious sign of an approaching attack may be the head pain itself. However, as they learn more about the condition, they may be able to detect some pre-pain signals, such as being overly talkative, having emotional changes or alterations in mental ability, craving specific foods and yawning. When recognized as migraine indicators, these may provide those few minutes of extra time which can be so helpful.

While it is not common, neither is it rare for victims to experience both "common" and "classic" migraine, the attacks varying from time to time.

SOME "UNCOMMON" MIGRAINES

In rare cases, migraine can be experienced as the pre-headache phenomena alone, impaired vision, flashing lights and so on, without any subsequent head pain. This is called *migraine equivalent* or, to some, "one-half of a migraine attack." Previously, it was not always easily diagnosed because of the absence of pain, and it can be both eerie and frightening for the victim, who can be expected to assume he is threatened by serious brain or vision problems. It is not uncommon for an ophthalmologist or optometrist to be the first to be visited. Fortunately such appointments usually lead to referrals since the absence of any actual eye problem often leads to a suspicion of migraine. It is not uncommon for *classic migraine* to occur periodically for many years until, in middle age, the headache component gradually fades, leaving only the pre-headache manifestations.

The pain of migraine can sometimes be experienced in areas of the body other than the head. In *abdominal migraine* a sufferer may experience the normal symptoms of common or classic migraine, except that an intense and debilitating pain is felt in the abdomen. Rarely the pain is experienced in the chest, leading to a diagnostic confusion with angina. Head pain may or may not accompany these chest and abdominal pains.

There is some evidence, yet to be confirmed by research, that in some teenage boys, migraine manifests itself as a sharp pain in the leg: the so-called *lower limb syndrome.* It often occurs following strenuous exercise or sports. The pain may be sudden and excruciating or it may last hours, sometimes interfering with sleep. Lower limb syndrome seems also to occur in girls, but, once again, the evidence is inconclusive.

In *retinal migraine* the pre-headache phase of an attack is characterized by partial or complete loss of vision in one eye. This can last for several minutes, and as vision returns, a dull pain generally begins behind the eye and spreads to the rest of the head.

Many migraine sufferers experience interference with their motor and speech abilities. (In some cases dizziness and clumsiness are very pronounced, and the syndrome is then categorized as *basilar migraine,* after the basilar artery, which supplies blood to the brain stem and the back part of the brain.) Handling of even small, light objects becomes difficult and clumsy, as does mere walking, and victims may find themselves bumping into things. Speech can become thickened and slurred, and the whole appearance is that of a person who is thoroughly drunk. In severe cases, the sufferer may even faint.

Temporary weakness of the eye muscles, causing double vision, is also often experienced in migraine, and the pupils may be of unequal size during an attack. If one pupil becomes greatly enlarged relative to the other and eye movements are impaired, the condition is called *ophthalmoplegic migraine* (indicating paralysis of the eye muscles).

Occasionally a migraine attack may be accompanied by a weakness in the arm and leg on one side of the body—a weakness which may approach complete paralysis. This may or may not be associated with a feeling of numbness or of pins and needles. This is *hemiplegic migraine* (indicating one-sided paralysis), and it may closely mimic the symptoms of stroke. The weakness usually clears up in an hour or so, though it can persist for days. If the weakness occurs on the right side of the body in a right-handed person, the brain's speech center may also be affected, making coherent conversation difficult or impossible. (A warning: women who suffer hemiplegic migraine should *never* take birth control pills. If they do, they run a high risk of these impairments becoming permanent. More will be said about this in Chapter 4.) Hemiplegic migraine tends to run in families, and this is one of the keys to its diagnosis. Roughly half of all of the children of an affected parent will also develop the condition. Because of the potential similarity to ominous medical matters, those with this type of migraine are doubly encouraged to wear some sort of identification such as a Medic-Alert bracelet.

Sometimes, tension headache *and* migraine are experienced. In some cases the tension headache triggers the migraine, through a mechanism which is not yet clearly understood. On other occasions, a tension headache may develop out of a migraine attack, as the sufferer contracts the muscles of the neck and shoulders in an attempt to keep pain-inducing movements of the head to a minimum. This condition is called a *mixed headache* in medical language, although sufferers will likely have their own, more colorful, descriptions.

MIGRAINE IN CHILDREN

Children and, sadly, even infants and toddlers can suffer migraine attacks of full-blown adult intensity. This was not generally recognized until recently, and the agitated behavior of children enduring the pain of migraine—behavior which may include banging the head on the floor or the side of the crib—was often mistakenly related to colic or temper tantrums. In fact, children make up more than 10% of the population of migraine sufferers.

While adults typically present an ashen appearance during an attack, children may also turn red or blue. Otherwise, the symptoms of migraine in children and infants are frequently the same as those in adults: principally, swelling of the hands and feet, corded veins, aversion to light and noise, nausea and vomiting and increased urination. Children, however, experience abdominal migraine more frequently than do adults.

Milder childhood migraine indicators usually consist of motion sickness, unpredictable stomach aches, and a propensity to vomit when excited—as during birthday parties or on departing in the family car on holidays. Such children used to be saddled with the label "highly strung." Parents who do not understand the nature of the condition are liable to find themselves trapped in a guilt-resentment scenario similar to that often experienced by the spouse of an adult sufferer. They may resent the inconvenience caused by the child's behavior and may admonish or even punish him—this followed by a generous dose of parental guilt. None of this, of course, does anybody any good.

A MIGRAINE ATTACK CHECKLIST

Common usage still refers to migraine as "a headache," but anyone who has suffered through AN ATTACK, whether it has lasted for hours, or days, knows that the total body is affected.

It is not unusual for victims to fail to mention symptoms that do not seem to be related to the head pain, not realizing that many of the symptoms they experience are "legal" and are, in effect, part and parcel of the migraine attack.

This is a simple checklist of some of the more common symptoms; fortunately, we have yet to encounter a sufferer who has had all of these!

Visual disturbances: double vision, difficulty in focussing, temporary or partial blindness, dazzling display of colored lights, spots or lines. Pages of print may have wavy lines, a hole in the middle or some lines darker than others. In some instances buildings, walls, television and even people may take on a pastel hue.

Dizziness.

Hallucinations: mild or not so mild, visual or otherwise.

Nausea: some may just feel queasy or uncomfortable.

Vomiting: may occur initially or may last some time.

Numbness and/or a tingling sensation: especially in the face, the shoulders, arms and hands and in the legs and feet, or down one side of the body.

Sensitivity to light, noise, aromas, tastes and certain textures.

Depression, irritability, tension and/or alteration in mood and outlook, often with a feeling of detachment. Others may experience feelings of extreme well being, of uncommon energy and vigor, as well as of excitement or expectation.

Frequent yawning: often an early sign of an approaching attack.

Unusual hunger: cravings for specific foods could be warning signs.

Talking: one can become aware of and be embarrassed by over-talkativeness, yet can do little about it. Difficulties may arise in forming words correctly. Some report that the tongue feels twice its normal size.

Mental abilities: difficulties often arise with respect to recall of frequently used words, of names, addresses and phone numbers. Many form their words or sentences backwards, so that the family or the physician has to decode the message.

Trembling: sometimes present to the point of making it next to impossible to hold a cup or glass.

Pain: initially felt in the head may, in time, extend to the neck, shoulders and arms and has been known, on some occasions, to travel to the chest area.

Blotchy patches: what looks like the beginning of a rash may appear. Veins may be seen and felt to be corded in the temple area but also in other parts of the body especially the arms and ankles. The unusual pallor (especially in children) may serve as a warning of an approaching attack.

Swelling: fingers and hands, as well as wrists, ankles, waists, breasts, legs may all swell. Often items of little weight, such as a pencil, simply fall from the hand, adding to one's frustrations.

Increased urination: insult added to injury.

Inability to think, to concentrate: the fact that an attempt to remember causes pain, is extremely unpleasant. Often one loses a degree of co-ordination so that the simple act of going through a door is hampered by the inability to judge distance resulting in bruised hips on many an occasion.

When the migraine attack is at its height there may be:

• pain in only one side of the head, or pain that has moved from one side of the head to the other, or from front to back.

• a feeling that one or both eyes are being pushed out of the head.

• there may also be present the feeling of tightness around the eyes, nose, and down to the mouth, jaw, teeth (often some swear every tooth needs to be pulled), some also note sore lips and tongue.

Some people experience relatively few of these symptoms while others will feel almost the whole arsenal of migraine effects on the body. These are all "legal" and are, contrary to what some feel, symptoms of the migraine itself. Of course all symptoms should be noted and reported to the examining physician.

THE DEMOCRATIC DISEASE

The fellowship of migraine is all-embracing. In the past, migraine sufferers were often consoled with the "fact" that they were of a group which was more intelligent, aware, sensitive, imaginative and artistic than the general run of the population. On the other hand, they have had attributed to them a lot of less attractive personality traits. A partial list of these, extracted from the medical literature, includes: perfectionism, rigidity, resentfulness, ambition, inflexibility, difficulty in handling repressed hostility or anger, a tendency to psychosexual conflicts, chronic depression, covert paranoia, deep-seated masochism, spitefulness, overt self-destructiveness and compulsive neatness and cleanliness.

One could easily infer from this set of subjective impressions a state of "repressed hostility" on the part of the practitioners responsible for the characterizations no less acute than that ascribed to their migrainous patients. The question is: "What scientific evidence is there for these characterizations?" The answer is: "None." In fact, rigidly controlled surveys of personality types among migraine sufferers have shown conclusively that the range of personality types present is no different than that found in the general population. Nonetheless, the myth of the migraine personality has shown powerful staying-power. The reason for this may lie partly in the fact that migraine sufferers who do happen to exhibit some of the compulsive neurotic traits of the "migraine personality" are likely to pay more frequent visits to their doctors and to be more demanding of them. Further, given the difficulty often experienced in diagnosing and successfully treating migraine, and the previous dearth of knowledge as to the precise mechanism of the condition, it is not difficult to see how a practitioner might grow to resent the insistent demands of a chronic patient. Doctors are human, too.

It is also evident that, while these unattractive traits may not be fixed or inborn personality defects in the sufferer, some of them may well develop as a superficial response to chronic pain and the continual disruption of daily life by often unpredictable pain. In fact, it would be surprising if a chronic sufferer did not become resentful, irritable and depressed on occasion. Most do.

The point of all of this is that, if a doctor sees these aspects of the "migraine personality" as causes of the problem rather than as effects of it, he may well find himself treating the wrong symptoms. He may, for example, prescribe tranquillizers in the belief that they will alter personality traits responsible in part for the migraine attacks when, in reality, these traits are not the roots but the branches. The eventual disappearance of the myth of the "migraine personality" will represent a significant step forward in the treatment of migraine.

A parallel myth associated with migraine sufferers has been that they come from the upper social strata—from the professional and managerial classes. The notion persisted for a couple of hundred years, bolstered, no doubt, by the frequency with which sufferers from "sick headache" turned up in romantic fiction and drama. Statistical studies carried out as recently as 1962 tended to reinforce the idea by showing a marked preponderance of "upper class" individuals among those visiting doctors because of headache. Later studies have demonstrated the obvious: poor people are less likely to spend the time and money required to pay a visit to a doctor for a non-lethal complaint than are rich people. The "lower classes" are therefore statistically under-reported in surveys of doctors. The fact is that migraine sufferers are distributed with admirable egalitarianism on every rung of the social ladder, from top to bottom.

Some epidemiological studies have spawned other myths about migraine. To verify the theory that migraine can result from doing finely detailed work indoors under artificial light, a study was made of a group of color retouchers in a printing plant. The verification was forthcoming; responses to the questionnaire handed around indicated a high incidence of migraine among the workers. But a later, more careful study contradicted the first. The problem lay in the wording of the first questionnaire. A large proportion of respondents to any question which suggests that they may be suffering from something will automatically agree. The original questionnaire had made such a suggestion.

It had been generally thought that the majority of migraine sufferers lived in urban centers as opposed to the quiet rural countryside. A single television program disproved this theory very quickly. Those who lacked delivery of a major daily newspaper or magazine heard, for the first time, of the existence of the Migraine Foundation via a trans-Canada television program prepared by the Canadian Broadcasting Corporation. It was rebroadcast three times; the mail response numbered in the thousands, and eight of every ten letters came from rural areas of Canada, the northern United States and into the Arctic. Without exception these non-urban listeners were literally starved for information.

There are no reliable statistics on the proportion of the population that suffers from migraine. But the estimates are constantly creeping upward as both the medical profession and the lay public gain a better understanding of the condition and how it may manifest itself. The estimate that is currently widely accepted is 20%.

Similarly, the economic cost of migraine is only beginning to be appreciated. People who suffer moderate to severe migraine lose an average of twenty-one working days a year: the average for all migraine sufferers is four days a year. (These figures apply to the United Kingdom, the United States, Canada and Scandinavia, and probably to most other industrialized nations.) In the United States, the cost to the economy of these lost working days has been estimated at eleven billion dollars a year.

The overwhelming weight of evidence now supports the contention that migraine is usually a genetic disorder and can thus be inherited. The exact mechanism of transference from one generation to the next is not well understood, but it seems likely that if both parents suffer from migraine, eight of every nine offspring will also have some degree of migraine at some point in their lives. A point to remember is that, though a person may be born migrainous, as few as three or four attacks a lifetime might be triggered, or as many as three or four a month or more, depending on what affects the individual. Further, about 80% of migraine sufferers report a family history of the condition. In cases where there is no apparent family history, the reason has sometimes been found to lie in inappropriate diagnosis and reporting of headache in parents, aunts, uncles, cousins and so on. They may have believed, for instance, that they suffered from tension or sinus headache.

Medical experiments have also shown that migraine and other headaches can be chemically induced in individuals who have no history of the condition. Sodium nitrite (a food preserva- tive), monosodium glutamate (a meat tenderizer and flavor enhancer used liberally especially in Chinese restaurants) and birth control pills have been specifically identified.

Migraine is more common among women than men, but how much more common is still uncertain. Attempts to establish a clear breakdown have been hampered by several factors, not the least of which is, in the current idiom, male "macho." Men are far less likely than women to seek professional help for their headaches, and, therefore, are less heavily reported in surveys. This undoubtedly has to do with cultural stereotypes in which migraine or "sick headache" is labelled as a woman's affliction. Men seem reluctant to ask for information on migraine even by mail. Our Migraine Foundation has found that three-quarters of all requests for information requested for male sufferers or sus- pected sufferers are, in fact, written by wives or daughters. Those requests that are written by men tend to volunteer far less information on the nature of the suspect headaches. Women correspondents will frequently describe their headaches in detail, but the typical format for male correspondence is: "Dear Sir or Madam: Please send me your kit on migraine. Thank you." It is not unusual for men who suffer from migraine while at work or in a social setting to ascribe the pain and nausea to a hangover—an affliction deemed to be more socially acceptable than migraine.

Early surveys which tended to ignore such cultural phenomena usually put the ration of female-to-male suffers at 75% to 25%. But more modern surveys put the proportions at 60% women and 40% men. There is some reason to believe that even this revised estimate may be somewhat conservative.

But whatever the final figures turn out to be, women will almost certainly outweigh men in the statistics to some degree. This is because women are susceptible not only to the conventional migraine triggers such as foods and weather changes, but also because their migraines can be triggered by hormonal changes occurring at puberty and during the menstrual cycle and at menopause. A common, though by no means universal, profile of migraine in women is for the headaches to begin with the onset of menstruation, to increase in frequency and intensity as the birth control pill is used, to decrease as the pill is discontinued, to disappear temporarily during pregnancy and then to reappear following childbirth. The headaches may again worsen during menopause and then disappear altogether. Because of this hormonal component in their condition, it is foolhardy for women who suffer from migraine to use the birth control pill as a method of contraception.

Just before moving on to a description of what happens in the body immediately prior to and during a migraine, it is worth repeating that migraine attacks people of both sexes and all ages, without regard to class, occupation or other social distinction. It is not a neurotic condition; it is an inherited disorder of the vascular system. There is no psychological profile or physical description of a "typical" migraine sufferer that holds up under close scrutiny, because there is no such thing as the "typical" migraine sufferer. The very number of people with migraine is proof enough of this—probably one in five of the people you know are victims in some degree, though many of them may never have had their condition properly diagnosed. Those who do understand the nature of the condition well enough to see through the miasma of myth and folklore surrounding it are well on the way to getting their headaches under control.

CHAPTER 3

Why it Hurts: Anatomy of a Headache

Despite decades of intensive research, there is still no clear and precise understanding of what goes on in the body during a migraine attack. The biochemical mechanism that results in the pain and discomfort of a typical attack has turned out to be extremely complex, and it will be some time before enough data can be collected to develop an explanation that will be accepted by all the experts.

Nevertheless, it is still possible to sketch in the bare outlines of the chain of events leading to the headache, given the understanding that the details of some of the linkages are still the subject of controversy among specialists.

We can begin with a statement that is *not* controversial: the pain of migraine is related to the stretching or dilation of blood vessels. Physicians who have carefully observed migraine sufferers have long suspected this, and it was shown to be the case in the middle of this century by Dr. Harold G. Wolff, an American who devoted much of his career to the study of head pain. Wolff's most convincing evidence came from a set of experiments conducted on volunteer migraine subjects. These were patients who were to undergo surgery for various reasons and who agreed to have it done under local anesthetic so that they could describe the sensations they felt as a result of various tests Wolff conducted. In one of these experiments, scalp arteries were exposed, and their walls were stretched by a clamp placed inside the artery. The volunteers were asked to describe their sensations: they said that it hurt. Wolff then attached threads to the artery walls and pulled rhythmically; the resulting sensation closely resembled the throbbing pain of migraine.

Interest then focussed on what caused the vessels to dilate in the first place. The logical place to begin such an investigation is in the analysis of the urine of migraine subjects during attacks. In due course it was discovered that a substance called *serotonin* was to be found in the body in abnormally high levels just prior to the head pain phase of a migraine attack, and that during the head pain itself, serotonin levels fell dramatically, to abnormally low concentrations. (Serotonin is so named because it was originally discovered in blood serum and because it gives resiliency or "tone" to vessel walls—hence, sero-tonin.)

Serotonin is an *amine*—one of a family of biological substances that regulate the functioning of the brain and blood vessels. Some amines are found in food, and others, like serotonin, are manufactured by the body by building blocks (amino acids) present in food. They can cause dilation and constriction of blood vessels, and they influence mood and behavior.

Once produced in the body, serotonin is stored in microscopic disc-shaped objects in the blood stream called platelets. Human blood contains anywhere from 200,000 to 400,000 of these platelets per cubic centimetre, and their chief function is to cluster together to form a clot whenever there is a puncture, cut or other breach of a blood vessel. When such a breach occurs, the platelets closest to the damage immediately stick to the walls of the vessel, and they release a substance into the blood which causes more platelets to congregate at the damage site. They also release serotonin, which acts to constrict the blood vessels in the area and thereby limit bleeding.

The platelets found in the blood of migraine subjects appear to have an enhanced ability to clump together to form a clot, and they also have the ability to release more serotonin than the platelets in the blood of non-migrainous subjects. Exactly why the blood platelets in migraine sufferers should have this characteristic is not yet understood.

Since serotonin acts as a constricting agent in large veins and arteries, there has been good reason to suspect that it plays an important role in migraine attacks. It is thought that the rise in serotonin during the pre-headache phase may result in a reduced blood flow to the brain, causing parts of it to malfunction in such a way as to produce visual, motor and speech disturbances. Then, when serotonin levels drop suddenly to abnormally *low* levels, blood vessels in the scalp rebound from their constricted state to become abnormally enlarged. Head pain follows.

There is other evidence to implicate this substance. The amine serotonin is known to prevent excretion of water from the body, and this could be the reason for the swelling of hands and feet that often precedes the head pain phase of migraine attacks. Serotonin also stimulates activity in the intestines, and this could account for the diarrhea often experienced as a pre-pain phenomenon. It has also been found that vomiting increases serotonin levels in the blood stream. This could explain why some migraine suffers find that their headaches are relieved or vanish altogether after vomiting: increased serotonin levels would act to constrict the painfully dilated vessels in the scalp. When serotonin is injected into the blood stream of someone suffering from a migrainous headache, the pain is usually alleviated. (Unfortunately, unpleasant side effects such as a tightness in the chest, flushing and "pins and needles" make serotonin unsuitable for routine treatment of migraine.)

Research which confirms that sexual arousal is often an accompaniment of migraine attacks may also serve to further implicate serotonin. Since this amine is known to have an inhibitory effect on the sex drive, it would be logical to expect arousal as its concentration in the blood falls during a migraine attack. And we now know that arousal does occur in a significant number of cases.

There are at least seven other so-called *vaso-active amines* which have the ability to dilate and/or constrict blood vessels, and recent research has implicated them as well in migraine attacks. These amines are adrenalin, noradrenalin, dopamine, octopamine, histamine, tyramine and beta-phenylethylamine. They are found in various foods which migraine subjects have identified as headache "triggers." Histamine, for example, is found in some cheeses and alcoholic drinks. Octopamine is found in some citrus fruits. Dopamine lurks in the broad bean, among other places. Beta-phenylethylamine is found in chocolate, cheese and alcoholic drinks. Tyramine (from *tiri,* the Greek word for cheese) is present in many cheeses. Ingestion of any or all of these foods will cause a headache in many migraine sufferers, and it appears to be the amines that do the trick.

But why should serotonin and other amines cause attacks in migraine sufferers and not headaches in other people? One explanation has been the suggestion that the blood vessels of migraine subjects have a tendency to overreact to the effects of vaso-active agents like these amines. That may be the answer, but it comes so close to over-simplication that it is of little or no use in the search for a solution to the problem. A more useful explanation has been provided by the unexpected side effects of a group of drugs that were in use for the treatment of severe depression. These drugs have the ability to inhibit the action of certain enzymes (biochemical catalysts) in the body known as *monoamine oxidase inhibitors* or MAO. When these were administered to mental patients suffering depression marked improvements resulted. But then reports began to be received of severe headaches developing when patients taking MAO inhibitors ate certain foods, especially cheese. Laboratory tests showed that the cheese contained a substance called tyramine, (one of the eight vaso-active amines) which was linked to the headpain.

Normally, tyramine is broken down in the body by MAO. This could not take place when the patient was using an MAO-inhibiting anti-depressant; hence the tyramine was able to act unhindered as a potent dilator of blood vessels, and a migrainous headache resulted. This fortuitously discovered chain of events has led some researchers to suspect that at the root of migraine there may lie a deficiency of some sort in the body's enzyme system—a deficiency which allows vaso-active amines to exert an improperly regulated and abnormally powerful influence in the bodies of migraine subjects. Why that influence should be felt almost exclusively in the vessels of one side or other of the head at a time is not understood.

Prostaglandins are another group of vaso-active substances which have recently come under close scrutiny in migraine research. As it turns out, these fatty acids have been inappropriately named; they were called prostaglandins because they were first discovered in semen and were thought to come from the prostate gland. However, it is now known that they occur in various parts of the bodies of both males and females.

Volunteers who had never experienced a migraine attack and who were injected with one of these prostaglandins quickly developed migraine-like symptoms, sometimes including even the visual disturbances of the pre-pain phase of classic migraine.

Another of the group of prostaglandins is thought to be released before menstruation to constrict the blood vessels supplying the lining of the uterus. If it turns out that the substance is released in other parts of the body as well, it could become a clue to unravelling the puzzle of "hormonal migraine" in women.

It is not difficult to see why specialists have difficulty in agreeing on a simple definition of migraine. It could be called an enzyme-based disorder, or a disturbance in the body's amine metabolism, or a vascular malfunction, or possibly some combination of all three.

Further complicating matters are those migraine attacks which seem to be entirely unrelated to foods containing vaso-active amines, or to any other external chemical "trigger." Some migraines seem to arise directly out of emotional stress; others are triggered by fasting; still others follow a sudden release from stress, as in the "weekend migraine" syndrome. Some are caused by a sudden drop in barometric pressure. There may yet be discovered some linkage between all of these various triggers and the body's enzyme and amine systems. In the case of stress-related migraines, for example, it may be that the headache is spawned by a release of adrenalin into the blood, which is a normal bodily reaction to stress. (Adrenalin is one of the vaso-active amines.) For the moment, the picture remains obscured by many questions that will only be answered through continued research.

There is another area of interest in all of this that begs for clarification. How does the dilation of blood vessels during a migraine cause pain? The same blood vessels dilate when the body gets overheated, or during exercise, but few sufferers get a migraine every time they have a hot bath or a game of squash. Some other agent must be at work.

The search for such an agent has led to the discovery that, during a migraine attack, there is an accumulation around the affected arteries in the scalp of a chemical irritant called *bradykinin*, which has a composition similar to that of wasp venom. Pure bradykinin is known to be a powerful pain-inducing substance. If you drain the fluid from a blister and then cut away the skin, a raw, sensitive area is exposed. If, after an hour or so you replace this same fluid over the tender area, it becomes very painful. Something has happened to the fluid in the test tube: in fact, a chemical reaction has taken place which has produced bradykinin.

Aside from its pain-producing qualities, bradykinin is also involved in the process of inflammation, which is part of the body's defence against infection. It lowers the pain threshold and adds to the dilation of affected blood vessels. All of these processes are consistent with what goes on in the body during a migraine attack.

Migraine sufferers sometimes feel as though parts of their scalp just below the skin are awash in acid, and this could be a result of the increased levels of bradykinin or related chemical irritants around the affected arteries.

Very little is known of the exact pathway followed by pain impulses travelling between the blood vessels and the pain-registering sections of the brain. Attempts at surgical alleviation of the pain of migraine by cutting various nerves have proved unsuccessful, indicating that several different pathways must be involved.

Once inside the brain, pain impulses can often be blunted by drugs, or by *endorphins,* the body's own pain killers. Endorphins are substances produced within the body which have a chemical make-up much like narcotic opiates such as codeine, morphine and heroin. Their release can be stimulated by stress, and it is thought that this may be one of the reasons why even severe injuries can, in some circumstances, fail to produce immediate pain—why soldiers, for example, can sometimes sustain terrible wounds and not notice them until the battle has ended.

There are strong indications that the amine serotonin, which has been linked to the dilation of blood vessels during migraine attacks, must be present in normal volume to ensure the full functioning of narcotic painkillers and of the body's own endorphins. This, apparently, accounts for the extreme severity of migraine pain (since serotonin levels are known to be abnormally low during the head pain phase of an attack) and for the fact that powerful drugs like codeine and morphine are often ineffective in relieving that pain. Many migraine subjects report that the narcotic drugs succeed in alleviating their suffering principally by putting them to sleep.

Just as a cure for migraine is unlikely as long as so many questions about its chemical and biological genesis remain unanswered, so it is unlikely as well that pharmacologists will be able to develop a truly effective drug to block the pain of migraine until the exact mechanism for the creation of that pain is understood.

Despite this, there is much that the sufferer can do right now to avoid migraine attacks and to relieve the pain and discomfort involved with those that cannot be avoided. These measures—preventive and therapeutic—are the subject of the next two chapters of this book.

CHAPTER 4

The Triggers and how to track yours down

Consider migraine as a gun: heredity loads it and points it at your head; the trigger causes it to fire. For several years, the Migraine Foundation in Toronto has been keeping careful records of migraine triggers reported by tens of thousands of correspondents and by the medical literature. They fall into four broad categories: dietary (by far the most common); hormonal (in the female population only); stress (both emotional and physical) and weather (especially sudden decreases in barometric pressure).

When all of the various triggers reported to affect the victims of migraine are catalogued as they are in the succeeding pages, the effect can be daunting, especially when it is realized that, in most cases, sufferers are affected by more than one trigger and that it often seems to take a combination of two or more triggers to set off the chemical chain reaction that results in an attack. Too often, sufferers will peruse such a list and decide that just about everything can trigger a migraine and that avoidance of triggers requires such a wrenching change in lifestyle that it is probably better to put up with the migraines.

It is therefore important to bear in mind that migraine is a very individualistic condition, and that triggers which act with sure-fire regularity on one sufferer may have no effect whatever on another. Even members of the same family may seldom be affected by the same triggers. The purpose of compiling an extensive list of the various triggers is simply to provide some idea of the kinds of factors involved, so that you will have somewhere to start in the process of tracking down your own.

Isolating those triggers that affect you requires patience and perseverance, but if you go about it systematically, you have the very worthwhile prospect of reducing the frequency and severity of your migraines by at least half. You may even be lucky enough to get rid of them altogether.

It may be that your particular trigger does not appear on our list. New and hitherto unsuspected mechanisms are reported to the Foundation with such regularity that our listings are incomplete almost as soon as they are compiled. Only a very few of the triggers reported to us can be validated scientifically: such tests are time-consuming and expensive. We normally consider a trigger to have been "authenticated" if it has been reported from five or more different sources, and in such cases the information is passed on to a medical advisory committee in the hope that one day soon research will isolate the precise chemical linkages involved. Sometimes, a search of the medical literature, or of our own computer filing system, will turn up the welcome information that the needed laboratory testing has already been done, or is currently underway. Our informal authentication process has proved remarkably reliable. An example: for several years, data thus compiled indicated strongly that diet played a much larger role in triggering migraines than that assigned to it in some of the medical literature. A recent two-year study by doctors at the National Hospital for Nervous Diseases and the Middlesex Hospital Medical School in Britain indicated that fully two-thirds of those sufferers involved in their experiments proved to be sensitive to certain foods and that eating those foods caused them to have attacks. On the other hand, our system has long indicated that stress is a far less significant factor in triggering migraine than has been believed by much of the medical profession: recent studies have gone a long way toward upholding that view as well.

KEEPING A LIST

One of the principal problems in systematically tracking down migraine triggers is that the body's reaction to foods consumed or events experienced can be delayed for twenty-four hours or more, depending on the sufferer's physical and/or mental condition at the time. This means that the *only* reliable way to isolate your triggers is to compile a list looking backward at least twenty-four hours from each migraine attack—a list in which is noted all relevant information: foods consumed, weather conditions, position in the menstrual cycle, unusual stress, sleeping habits, timing of meals and snacks, time of day, duration and intensity of the attack and so on. Experience has shown that, unless you are one of the very rare sufferers whose attacks occur every day, it is best not to keep a daily record of such information but, rather, to compile it on a "per attack" basis. Daily records tend to become discouragingly unwieldy and complex.

When several of these lists have been compiled, a comparison of them will often reveal a pattern in which one or more trigger mechanisms stand out quite clearly. It may be a specific sleeping pattern, such as sleeping in on weekends; it could be something in the diet, or a skipped meal, or a hostile outdoor or indoor environment, or recurring stress or perhaps a combination of two or more factors. Once such a pattern is observed, each suspected trigger must be isolated and avoided to determine whether the headaches persist in its absence. Of course, some triggers, such as hormonal changes and fluctuations in barometric pressure, are impossible to avoid. However, it may be that these "unavoidable" triggers are effective only when acting in concert with other trigger mechanisms. Once these other mechanisms have been eliminated, the duration and intensity, if not the frequency, of the headaches may be substantially reduced. They may even be eliminated.

Years ago I developed a kind of point system for myself based on my subjective reaction to various migraine triggers. It began one day when I was unable to pin down exactly what had triggered an attack. After writing down everything that had occurred that day, a picture emerged:

	Points
Insufficient sleep	100
Rushed through breakfast—ate too little	150
Drove through heavy morning traffic to meet executive at airport	150
Morning sun in eyes while driving—forgot sun glasses	300
Drove 150 miles with talkative passenger	50
Quiche Lorraine for lunch (contains cheese)	100
White wine with lunch	150
Outdoor meeting—sat in afternoon sun	200
Afternoon coffee	100
Longer than five hours between lunch and dinner	300
Drive back into city—into setting sun (bought sun glasses)	250
Late committee meeting, sipped glass of white wine	150
Late to bed—too tired to have snack	250 +
Total:	2,250

As a rule, a total of one thousand to twelve hundred points can trigger a migraine for me.

There is no scientific or medical basis for the assigning of points to the various trigger mechanisms—only my own forty years of experience with migraines. Other sufferers will have different assessments. Still, compiling such a list helped me to understand how my own migraines might be triggered on those days when there is no single, obvious cause such as a rapid drop in barometric pressure or the onset of menstruation.

COMMON TRIGGERS

Mental and Emotional Stress

More often the cause of tension headaches than of migraines, mental and emotional stress are, nonetheless, direct trigger mechanisms in a significant number of cases. Moreover, migraines are frequently triggered by tension headaches which can result from stress. It should be borne in mind that stress arises not only out of unhappy or painful experiences, but also out of joy, excitement and surprise as well.

In our surveys of thousands of migraine sufferers over the years, we have found that a great many of them list stress and tension as the prime triggers of their headaches. We now believe that many of them do so mistakenly, partly because the conventional wisdom about migraine says that it is strictly a stress-related condition.

Unless you live an exceptionally placid life, if you begin with the assumption that stress *must* be involved, it is never difficult to find an example of it somewhere in the twenty-four hours preceding an attack and to see it as a trigger. We have shown to our own satisfaction, through some informal experiments, that it was being over-reported. Whenever there is a rapid drop in barometric pressure in the Toronto region, the Foundation is inundated with telephone calls from migraine sufferers who want to know what is causing their headaches and what they can do to obtain relief. On a Monday following a weekend during which there had been a precipitous drop in pressure, we responded to the inquiries of our first twenty callers with a question that contained a suggestion: we asked them all whether they felt that any unusual stress might be involved in their attacks of the previous weekend. Nineteen of the twenty replied positively that, on reflection, there had been some stress over the weekend. Only one self-assured individual adamantly ruled out stress or tension. We followed up these calls by asking the sufferers to keep charts of possible triggers for the twenty-four hours prior to their subsequent attacks. Eventually, a majority of those twenty callers were able to distinguish a clear relationship between their attacks and either large or relatively small declines in barometric pressure. The scenario was repeated one Monday following Mother's Day. Most of our callers felt that family stress was to blame for their attacks: they had not taken into consideration the low barometric pressure that had come with the heavy rainfall that Sunday.

Those who are able with certainty to ascribe their migraine attacks to stress are, in a sense, fortunate. Stress and its treatment is a field in which there has been a virtual explosion of information in recent years. There are now several excellent books on the subject, and many kinds of stress-relieving and stress-avoiding therapies have been newly developed or adapted from older ideas.

Many people find that it is not stress, but the release from it (stress come-down) that triggers their migraines. The so-called weekend migraine syndrome has been well documented for years, but, until recently, it was thought to arise out of the "migraine personality." Since all migraine sufferers are compulsive, perfectionist and "workaholic," the reasoning went, the weekend migraine must be a subconsciously-induced reaction to being away from work. The reasoning has a fatal flaw, of course, in that there is no such thing as a "migraine personality."

Nobody knows exactly why the transition from stress to relaxation should trigger migraines. But we do know that attacks can often be avoided by making the switch a gradual one. Sleeping in beyond an extra hour is to be avoided absolutely. Most of us are aware that if we sleep in too long, we will arise groggy, irritable and generally out-of-sorts, and, normally, this will mean that a migraine is on the way. The outcome is often the cancellation of a planned weekend outing: the resulting strain on family relationships does nothing to alleviate the problem. If you are subject to migraine on the weekend, *do not sleep in.*

Physical Stress

Light: Strong direct or reflected light, or rapidly changing light patterns can trigger migraines in many people. Where the problem is the sun's glare, whether on snow, on city streets, on water or sand, light-polarizing sun glasses are the obvious answer.

Some people find night driving a problem: the headlights of oncoming traffic, the painted road markings flashing by, the lighted signs and the streetlights combine to trigger an attack.

Most migraine sufferers find that fluorescent lights are impossible to endure during an attack, and many report that they can also trigger attacks. The problem is greatly magnified if the lights are working improperly and are flickering.

Movies and television (especially color television) can trigger migraines if the viewer is exposed to very rapid changes in light patterns, or to rapid camera movement. And, of course, for those who are sensitive to the assaults of light and sound, discotheques might have been designed deliberately as migraine factories. Definitely off-limits. As are clothing stores and boutiques of the modern genre, with their strobe lights and pulsating music.

Some years ago it was brought to our attention at the Foundation that professional hockey players of the National Hockey League (NHL) often suffered from migraine attacks during or just after a game. Many of the players had been told that their headaches arose out of the stress and anxiety of the game. However, for some professionals of vast experience, this did not seem to be an adequate answer. Careful observation revealed that their suspicions were largely correct. The problem was found to lay principally in the glare of arena lights on the ice surface and the intense concentration on the small black puck gliding over that surface. Migraines during and after practice sessions were less frequent, apparently because lighting was normally relatively subdued in the absence of the television cameras which were there to broadcast the scheduled games.

About that same time we were asked to answer another intriguing question: why was it that bus drivers seemed to have a far higher incidence of migraine attacks than the subway or underground drivers employed by the same transit authority? Here again, simple observation provided an answer. The bus driver's position ahead of the vehicle's front wheels exposed him to the glare of sunlight reflected off the cars around him.

Light-polarizing sunglasses solved the problem for some; but for others, the headaches persisted. More observation brought with it the realization that bus drivers are routinely exposed to heavy doses of exhaust fumes, particularly in heavy stop-and-go traffic. The ultimate solution for migrainous bus drivers proved to be a request for a transfer to the subway system.

Noise and vibration: Many sufferers report that noise can trigger their attacks: the trouble is that, what is noise to one person's ears is music to another's. We heard of one interesting therapeutic use of sound that always makes us smile—the young matron who, when she feels a migraine approaching, takes her prescribed medicine, dims the lights, elevates her head, dons well-cushioned ear phones and puts Beethoven on the stereo. But only Beethoven. "No other composer eases the migraine," she claims.

Noise need not be very loud and/or continuous to trigger an attack: the bedlam created by a few dozen kids in an indoor swimming pool; the low-frequency thump thump thump of the neighbor's loudspeakers; the pneumatic drill ripping up the street outside your window—that sort of noise will do the trick.

Perhaps there is a clue to the kinds of noise that most offend in the experience of classic migraine sufferers who notice strange auditory effects during the attack. Normal, usual sounds such as traffic or people talking as they walk along the street seem dull and muffled, as if a layer of custard had been poured over everything. Yet through this strange melange of muffled sound, a sharp noise like the honking of a car horn or the screech of tires will penetrate like a white-hot ice pick, causing excruciating pain.

Noisy, vibrating household appliances such as vacuum cleaners can also trigger attacks.

Microwave ovens: Low-level radiation from these appliances can trigger migraine attacks and can cause headaches in non-migrainous people. Problems with radiation leakage are rare, particularly with post-1974 models if the seal around the door is inspected frequently and kept clean by regular wiping with a dampened cloth. Users are warned not to place any metal object in the metal mesh on the door while the oven is in operation: it could act as an antenna and radiate microwaves outside the oven. Naturally, those who use the ovens most frequently are most susceptible, notably waitresses and those who serve in fast-food outlets, bars, pubs and so on. If you suspect that a microwave oven may be causing problems for you, have it tested for leakage. This sort of testing is frequently done free of charge by national or local government agencies. If this is not the case where you live, the best bet might be to contact a local consumers' organization to ask for advice.

Odors, aromas and smells: The more intense and penetrating the odor, the greater the effect. For many, the odor of fresh paint will trigger an attack. If you are planning to redecorate, test a small area first to see if the smell can be handled, or if you're going to need alternative accommodations until the stuff has completely dried. For some, many solvents and cleaning compounds will also trigger attacks though it is sometimes possible with diligent searching to find a product whose odor can be tolerated. In some cases, a combination of triggers might be involved—for instance, using a cleaning compound while bending over or stooping.

Non-smokers and, sometimes, even smokers often report that second-hand smoke will trigger an attack, particularly in poorly ventilated surroundings.

Some sufferers report that attacks can be triggered by specific perfumes, but there seems to be no clear pattern. Others report being affected by a whole family of perfumes, such as those based on musk oil. It is quite common for sufferers to be affected by specific scents found in cosmetics, soaps, shampoos, rinses, hair sprays, deodorants and room deodorizers, but, once again, there is no pattern evident in the complaints. The odor trigger mechanism seems to be more personal than most.

Cooking odors: Cooking odors are seldom pungent enough to actually trigger a migraine attack, but they may be sufficient to put a sensitive sufferer off his feed, so that he or she skips a meal. And this, of course, can lead to a fasting migraine.

Steam: This is often a trigger for housewives and others who work over stoves and ovens on the festive days that put a heavy emphasis on food: Christmas, Hannukah, Thanksgiving. The continuous blasts of steam encountered as the contents of the many pots on the stove are tested, or as the oven door is opened for basting operations, along with the generally high humidity this creates in the kitchen, can trigger a migraine attack. Such attacks are frequently and erroneously attributed to family tension, to excitement or to stress related to the holiday.

Hot tubs, hot baths, saunas and steam baths are all to be treated warily by the sufferer who is sensitive to steam.

Poor ventilation: Workers in modern office towers are often subject to migraine, frequently at about three o'clock in the afternoon. The chances of a migraine developing are increased if one stays inside the building all day, without taking a breathing spell outside. Again, nobody knows exactly why sealed office towers and their conditioned air should trigger migraines, although some suspect it may have to do with an imbalance in the charged particles in the air—a lack of negative ions. Experiments have been carried out using negative ion generators in conjunction with a building's air conditioning system, and these have been encouraging. The high cost of the generators has, unfortunately, limited their use, particularly in North America.

Television studios are notorious breeding grounds for migraine, and it is not only the bright lights that are to blame, for the crew behind the cameras (and the lights) are just as susceptible as the on-camera personalities. Here too, the principal trigger seems to be related to the sealed atmosphere. A five-minute break outside the studio each hour can be a substantial help in reducing the frequency of migraine attacks.

Motion: Motion sickness in children is often a sign that they are migrainous and will develop migraine attacks later in life.

We've received reports from adult sufferers who cannot sit in the front seat of a moving car without developing a migraine, but who are fine if they ride in the back. (We have also received a report from one man who cannot ride in the back seat but is comfortable in the front.)

Rocking chairs and beds and chairs which offer vibration can also lead to nausea, if not full-blown attacks, in migraine sufferers. Some sensitive subjects find it impossible to talk with anyone who is rocking back and forth in a chair, without becoming nauseous.

A sufferer from mild migraine can frequently handle the gentle motion of a ship, but others have no sea legs whatever.

The real testing ground for this trigger is the circus midway with its death-defying rides. Try one, and you may end up seriously ill. This is something to keep in mind especially if a migrainous child is among your charges.

Shock: Even a mild blow to the head can result in a migraine in some sufferers. This particular trigger may run in families: one specialist has noted it in the father and son in one family and in one adult and two children in another. The migraine attack usually follows the shock of a blow by about twenty minutes. This trigger is of course especially prevalent among those who are involved in sports like football, boxing, lacrosse, hockey and so on, where it is not unusual for the head to receive a severe jolt. The vomiting and severe head pain which accompany the migraine thus triggered can closely mimic the effects of brain damage and have been known to cause understandably serious, though unwarranted, concern among coaches and parents of young athletes. However, even if there is a history of migraine, it is advisable to have an immediate medical check up.

Teeth and occlusion: One of the many problems of living with migraine is sorting out which symptoms are migraine-related, and which indicate the existence of some unrelated medical problem. Dental problems are a case in point. Migraine attacks will sometimes cause pain in the upper and lower jaws, and even in the gums. On the other hand, the pain of a toothache can sometimes be referred by the nervous system to other areas of the head, and such pain can also trigger a migraine attack.

Ill-fitting dentures and plates can trigger migraine attacks.

When the bite is out of adjustment because of the loss of molars on one side of the mouth, the stress of chewing on one side only can result in pain felt in the ear and temple: this can trigger a migraine attack, or it can be intensified during an attack caused by some other trigger in a migrainous person.

If the hinge between the upper and lower jaws (the tempero-mandibular joint which can be felt just in front of the ear) is put out of alignment during surgery or in an accident or because of some dental problem, the resulting pain can trigger recurrent migraines. Often the problem evolves gradually as a result of years of teeth-clenching and grinding: it becomes obvious when a clicking is felt or heard with each bite.

If migraine pain, therefore, seems often to travel down into the jaw area, your neurologist may refer you to a specialist in problems of the jaw who will likely be affiliated with the Society for Temporo-mandibular Occlusion. A painless test can be done with an instrument that graphically illustrates what is going on as the jaw joints are used. Often, the malocclusion can be corrected simply and painlessly.

Each year the Migraine Foundation hears from several people who have been helped in this way. For some, the malocclusion was the primary migraine trigger so that, upon correction, the frequency and intensity of their attacks changed dramatically. With others, the degree of relief has been less significant, indicating that the malocclusion was not the main cause of their migraines.

Hypertension: One of the most frequent misunderstandings between doctor and patient reported to us arises out of a diagnosis of hypertension. Often, the patient will interpret this to mean "hypertense," when, in fact, it is merely medical jargon for high blood pressure. Another, similar misunderstanding can occur when a doctor refers a migraine sufferer to a neurologist for diagnosis and/or treatment. An irate patient contacted us to complain that his doctor had failed to understand the nature of his condition, had apparently concluded that he was a "nervous type" and had referred him to a neurologist to have his "nerves" investigated. We explained that a neurologist is a specialist in disorders of the body's nervous system, and not in "nerves" as in "I feel nervous."

Headache is not normally a symptom of high blood pressure. A small percentage of those who suffer from this condition may experience a slight headache on awakening in the morning, or, less frequently, in moving from a prone or sitting position to standing. However, this usually disappears as soon as one is up and about and is soon forgotten.

But hypertension in migraine victims may lead to an increase in the frequency of attacks, an aggravation which will be removed with diagnosis and subsequent control of the high blood pressure. Have your blood pressure checked at least once a year.

Exercise: Exercise which serves to tone up the cardiovascular system can be beneficial, but the form must be carefully chosen by those who suffer from frequent and severe migraines. Sports which involve bodily contact and where there is a risk of receiving an occasional blow to the head can cause problems, as can sports which involve a lot of rapid eye movement and concentration on a small object: tennis and badminton are two examples. Jogging is very frequently reported as a trigger of migraine attacks, though men with "cluster" have reported benefits. In some cases, almost any exercise which involves bending or stooping in a head-down position can bring on an attack.

Sexual intercourse: This, too! After the first few reports of migraine developing during or immediately after sexual intercourse reached the Foundation, we made a thorough check of the medical literature. Where intercourse was mentioned as a trigger, it was almost without exception qualified as "rare" or "uncommon." Since that time, our own listing of such reports have grown to such an extent that we are led to believe this problem is considerably more common than had been thought. Sufferers who are reluctant to discuss their sex-related head-aches with their physician will often unburden themselves to a stranger whom they know to be a fellow sufferer, and that often means the person on the other end of the phone at the Migraine Foundation. In some cases, an understanding spouse has been the one to initiate contact. Both men and women are affected.

Dramatic cardiovascular changes occur during intercourse (and during masturbation): in a normal person, these may combine with emotional excitement and contraction of the muscles in the neck, jaw and shoulders to produce a tension headache sometimes referred to as a benign sex headache. In migraine sufferers this, combined perhaps with the sudden increase in blood pressure and consequent dilation of blood vessels that occurs during intercourse, can trigger a migraine attack, generally at or shortly after climax. The resulting head-aches vary greatly in duration, from a few minutes to several hours. The attacks appear to be unrelated to such considerations as coital position, activity or passivity, or length of foreplay.

We do know that the very knowledge that others suffer from the same problem has helped to relieve the understandable psychological pressure that can build up through ignorance of the facts.

Some physicians suggest that a vaso-constricting medica-tion be taken fifteen to twenty minutes before intercourse. What is sacrificed in the spontaniety of the moment is regained in an ability to enjoy the afterglow.

Tight clothing: Tight collars and waistbands, hats, wigs and so on can all cause discomfort leading to a migraine. Most sufferers choose their wardrobe carefully with an eye to comfortable, easy fit.

Hormonal Migraine

Specialists estimate that more than 60% of women who suffer migraine regularly have attacks related to their menstrual cycle. In light of our experience at the Migraine Foundation, I would be willing to go beyond that to state that if hormonal migraine did not exist, the ratio of male to female migraine sufferers would be close to fifty-fifty, as opposed to the actual rather large female predominance.

Menstrual migraine: Before getting into the links between menstruation and migraine, it may be useful to review briefly what happens to the body during menstruation. Each month, the female reproductive system prepares itself to harbor a fertilized egg or ovum. At the beginning of each cycle (which is arbitrarily taken to be the onset of menstrual bleeding), the pituitary gland, a small organ at the base of the brain, secretes substances which are carried by the blood stream to the ovaries, and which stimulate the production of eggs or ova. At the same time, the ovaries are stimulated to produce the hormone estrogen, one function of which is to help prepare the uterus to receive a fertilized egg. One of the eggs produced by the ovaries develops more than the others and at mid-cycle (roughly the fourteenth day) it leaves the ovary and descends to the uterus. As this occurs, the estrogen level in the blood falls markedly. Within a day or two, the ovaries begin producing a second hormone, progesterone, and new supplies of estrogen. During the rest of the second half of the cycle, production of both of these hormones increases, continuing the preparation of the lining of the uterus to receive a fertilized egg. If the egg is in fact fertilized by sperm, it proceeds to implant itself in the uterus. But if the egg is not fertilized by about the twentieth day of the cycle, the ovaries shut down production of both estrogen and progesterone, causing the lining of the uterus to slough, producing the menstrual flow.

A Persian poet—a male Persian poet—once described this flow as the weeping of an empty womb.

Most authorities now believe that menstrual migraine is

related directly to hormonal changes during the cycle. Some relate the trigger mechanism to declines in estrogen levels, while others believe the connection lies in the ratio of estrogen to progesterone in the system. Attacks usually come just before the menstrual flow begins, when estrogen and progesterone production ceases in the ovaries. Often, the attack(s) will ease once the flow starts. Other experience attacks throughout the first day or so when the flow is heaviest. Still others experience a constant low-level migraine throughout their period. In both cases, a severe attack may develop on the last day of the menstrual flow, or on the following day. Some women have noted that attacks may also occur regularly at mid-cycle, during ovulation, when estrogen production falls off briefly.

Some physicians, believing that water retention during the menstrual cycle produces headaches, prescribe diuretics or water pills. While these may make a woman more comfortable in a general sense, they seem to do little to prevent or ease menstrual migraine attacks.

Not all headaches occurring at the time of menstruation are migraines. Those who experience emotional ups and downs during menstruation may develop tension headaches. These are easily differentiated from migraine, and should be treated for what they are.

Any form of head pain connected with menstruation is unnatural: it is not a normal part of the hormonal cycle. Those who experience blockbuster headaches *must* have the matter investigated, because nowhere is it written, not even in Persian poetry, that women shall put up with headaches during menstruation.

Hormonal migraine can be a crippling problem, and some women have sought rather extreme solutions—even hysterectomies. Hormonal injections which counteract the natural hormonal fluctuations in the body perhaps ought to provide relief, but have had little success to date. The main problem is that there is no way of knowing what combination or amount of hormones is just right. Every now and then, through sheer luck, a physician may hit upon the right pill or injection at the right time for the right patient. What is far more likely to happen is that the hormone treatment will aggravate the existing migraine problem, or cause other hormonal side effects. Better odds are offered at the race track.

Hysterectomies became quite popular as a treatment for menstrual migraine during the 1930s, but the results were disappointing. About one in ten thousand women indicated that they felt the operation had helped, and, even in these cases, there is no certainty that the migraines were not being triggered by some other medical condition which was coincidentally helped by the hysterectomy. The pain of the operation, the scars, the occasional complications, the period of recuperation plus the fact that the operation had not relieved the migraine problem were all bad enough; but most disappointing of all for many women was the fact that the migraines continued on the same cycle as before, ending only when the body would have gone through menopause in the natural course of events. Sometimes you just can't fool Mother Nature.

Puberty and menopause are times of great hormonal changes in women, and, as one would expect, there are usually changes in migraine patterns. Puberty often marks the beginning of true migraine in children who previously had experienced only mild symptoms such as motion sickness, or no symptoms at all. At menopause, many women experience a brief flare-up in their attacks followed by a welcome decrease in their frequency and severity. They often disappear completely.

If you experience hormonal migraine only, the chances of improvement with menopause are better than 50%. However, many woman are affected by triggers other than, or in addition to, hormonal fluctuations. While the hormonal migraines may fade or disappear, there is no guarantee that the others will similarly ease or vanish.

Hormonal supplements are frequently prescribed for women who have lost their natural supplies through menopause (or hysterectomy where the ovaries have been removed). Often there are excellent reasons why such hormonal supplements may be welcome and necessary. Severe menopausal symptoms such as hot flushes, perspiration, depression and so on may disrupt family life and career and ought to be brought under control.

However, some women develop migraine for the first time, or experience a worsening of an existing migraine condition after beginning such medication. The decision as to whether or not to continue with the hormone supplements in such cases boils down to a trade-off between symptoms: which are the most bearable, is the question that must be answered.

Migraine and the pill: The contraceptive pill can also cause problems. Made up of varying combinations of estrogen- and progesterone-like hormones, the pill alters the hormonal balance of the body so as to prevent pregnancy. Many women with a family history of migraine report that their first attacks occurred on beginning to take the pill. What is more disturbing is the fact that women who have no family history of migraine have also begun having attacks when the pill has been prescribed. A number of government health departments have now begun circulating warnings recommending that the pill not be prescribed for those with a family history of classic migraine or an existing classic migraine condition. There is a growing suspicion that women with classic migraine who take the pill run an increased risk of stroke.

If common migraines develop or increase in severity, the physician may consider switching his patient to a pill containing a lower dosage of estrogen. If that does not help, another form of birth control is indicated.

Many specialists believe that if common migraine problems arise with the pill, its use should be totally discontinued within eighteen months of its initial use. Otherwise, there is a risk of the change in migraine patterns becoming constant, the "damage" being, to a great extent, irreversible.

Migraine and pregnancy: This brings us (though not inevitably) to pregnancy and childbirth, two more periods in a woman's life when hormonal changes occur. During pregnancy, about 80% of women find that their migraines either diminish in frequency and severity, or disappear altogether. For some, this blessing covers the entire nine months; for others, it begins at the end of the first three months, and, for still others, it does not begin until six months into the pregnancy. Often, the improvement will continue throughout the period of lactation as well, which is as good a reason as any for breast-feeding. The migraines usually return once pregnancy and lactation are over. For the other 20% of women, the pattern may be, unfortunately, entirely different. Some report that their migraines not only continue throughout pregnancy but that they become more frequent and/or severe— and this new pattern persists beyond the end of lactation. A small number report that an almost continuous nine-month migraine must be endured.

It is advisable to stop taking all migraine medication (and, for that matter, any non-vital medication, prescription or non-prescription) as soon as pregnancy is confirmed or even suspected. Then, of course, you should consult with your physician.

This may be a problem for those women who continue to experience migraines during part or all of their pregnancy. Occasionally, a physician will agree to limited and careful use of a mild migraine medication after the important first few months of the fetus's development, but, ideally, the less medication used, the better. It is at this time that many women seek therapy which does not involve medication, the most common being bio-feedback training and self-hypnosis, as taught by physicians or other qualified practitioners. (Both of these techniques can also be useful during childbirth—an added bonus.)

The pattern of migraine can change from one pregnancy to the next. We have spoken with women who had such a miserable time with migraine during their first pregnancy that they seriously considered not having a second child. In most cases they went ahead anyway and were delighted to find the pattern had changed.

Some women report that their first experience with migraine came following a pregnancy. This, apparently, is because the dramatic hormonal changes involved served to bring an existing migraine condition to the surface where it could be recognized as such.

While it does not happen to all migrainous women, it is not uncommon for a severe migraine to be experienced somewhere around the third or fifth day after childbirth, particularly if the baby is not being breast-fed. If you are still in hospital, you may have difficulty in getting migraine medication in time unless you have made explicit arrangements in advance with your doctor and the supervising nurse. On returning home from the hospital, you may not have your migraine medication on hand, or else during the long holiday from migraine provided by pregnancy, the expiry date on the medicine may have run out. It could be wise to have your prescription filled and ready, but do discuss this with your physician. Medication should be questioned if you are breast-feeding.

Weather Migraine

Barometric pressure: Many migraine victims are sensitive to changes in barometric pressure, often coming down with an attack whenever the mercury falls much below 30.0 inches (101.6 kPa). That fact was never more in evidence than on January 26, 1978, when a major blizzard immobilized much of eastern Canada and the northeastern United States. The low pressure area that accompanied the storm caused barometers to dip to the lowest levels recorded in 140 years. Beginning two days before the storm arrived in full force, our telephones at the Migraine Foundation were ringing almost constantly: thousands of people were being affected by migraines so severe that some feared for their lives. During a more recent and less dramatic period of very low barometric pressure, we received a call from a physician who wondered if we had any idea why all of his migraine patients had trooped into his office one by one during the preceding day or two, seeking relief from severe pain. So predictable is the effect of low barometric pressure on migraine sufferers that it would probably be possible to predict weather by monitoring the number of calls going through the Foundation telephone system.

Some of these callers recognize the connection between the migraines they are experiencing and the unusual atmospheric conditions. Many, however, do not. Some believe their migraine medications are no longer effective; some feel their migraines "have reached a dangerous stage," and still others fear their migraines have been superseded by a life-threatening condition of some sort—perhaps a brain tumor.

In most cases, the only help we are able to offer our callers is an explanation of the relationship between barometric pressure and migraine, an assurance that they are not alone in their suffering and whatever up-to-date information we have from the weather office on the likely duration of the low pressure conditions. People being what they are, most are grateful for even that cold comfort.

The treatment of weather migraine is extremely difficult because the triggering mechanism may remain in place for days, even weeks on end, and the migraine will persist for as long as the trigger is there. A vaso-constricting medication (ergotamine) taken at the onset of an attack may hold it off for a few hours; but the drug will eventually wear off, and, with the trigger mechanism still in place, the migraine will recur. Continuous use of these drugs is inadvisable for several reasons (See Chapter 6), and, in any case, they do not seem to be very effective where low barometric pressure is the trigger. Analgesics may erase the pain, but only if taken in doses too large even to contemplate. Even narcotics administered under medical supervision will provide only a few hours of relief, and at the end of that time, the pain will be back in full force.

Not all episodes of low pressure are long-lived. Sometimes a summer storm will sweep in, unload its rain amid a cacophony of thunder and be gone within the space of a couple of hours, leaving blessed relief from headache in its wake. And, sometimes, the barometric pressure will fluctuate rapidly, so that no sooner has one migraine attack eased than another is on its way.

The precise details of the linkage between barometric pressure and migraine are still under investigation. However, it is known that, under normal conditions, the pressure within our bodies and the atmospheric pressure outside are in equilibrium. If they were not we would either explode like an over-inflated balloon, or be crushed under the weight of the tons of air bearing down on us from above. When the atmospheric pressure falls and the barometer goes down, that equilibrium is disturbed, and the pressure inside the body is slightly higher than that outside. This results in an outward expansion of the gases and liquids within the body. The arteries of the brain and scalp appear to be very sensitive to changes of this sort: blood vessels become dilated and a migraine attack results.

Those who are especially sensitive are frequently affected by storm systems passing twenty or thirty miles distant; but their attacks will generally be less severe in such cases than if they were in the direct path of the bad weather. A quarter-century ago Hurricane Hazel cut a swath of terrible destruction and loss of life across southern Ontario: on its twenty-fifth anniversary we polled a group of migraine sufferers who remembered the storm, asking them where they lived at the time and how they would describe their migraine attacks (if any) during the storm. We matched the results with a map of the course of the hurricane. The results dovetailed exactly: those who had suffered "excruciating" attacks had been in the direct path of the storm; those who had "severe" attacks were on the periphery, often as far as fifty or sixty miles away.

The nature of barometric fluctuations varies according to geography: in some arid regions they are quite moderate and infrequent, while on sea coasts and near large bodies of water they can be frequent and extreme. Another, much larger, survey undertaken by the Foundation confirmed that people moving from one geographic region to another generally notice a distinct change in the patterns of their migraines (if they suffer from weather migraines).

This raised a slightly frivolous question in our minds—we wondered if there was any place on earth where a sufferer might spend a few weeks with the assurance that the barometer would remain high and stable. We asked our local weather experts, and, after several days, they provided us with two such locations: the middle of the Dead Sea and the bottom of the Grand Canyon. We now have frequent visions of Grand Canyon health spas and Dead Sea pleasure cruises.

Because atmospheric pressure varies with altitude (falling as altitude increases and the column of air above us becomes shorter) some migraine sufferers find it difficult to spend much time in very tall buildings.

It also means that almost all those who are sensitive to low barometric pressure find long-distance flight a problem. (Short hops are easier to tolerate because the aircraft do not reach high altitudes.) This includes both cabin crew and flight attendants on commercial airliners. Some migrainous passengers and crew members may experience attacks during flight, as soon as the aircraft reaches high altitude (about 35,000 feet, some report). Others don't feel the effect until shortly after descent or landing.

Where classic migraine is involved, it has been reported that the visual, aural and other disturbances of the pre-headache phase will disappear if oxygen is administered. The headache phase, however, remains unchanged.

When the Migraine Foundation was established, we began receiving many inquiries from people who were reluctant to discuss their problem with family or company physicians, for fear that this might affect their job status. High on the list were police officers and pilots and other flight-crew members. Pilots reported an unusually high percentage of classic as opposed to common migraine attacks. None of them expressed any concern about being able to competently pilot the aircraft during the head pain itself; all felt that this presented little problem. What did concern them was the unpredicatability of the visual disturbances accompanying the pre-headache phase of a classic attack. We should point out that only a few of the pilots we spoke to flew large commercial passenger aircraft: most flew military planes, or executive jets or charter aircraft operating in northern oil and gas fields.

Some of the commercial pilots who had, through seniority, been assigned to long-distance flights, chose voluntarily to revert to the short-hop low-altitude milk runs. Others, after consulting with specialists, learned to take vaso-constricting medication at the first sign of an attack, to wear polarizing sun glasses and, most important, to let the co-pilot take over until the aura and its visual disturbances had passed.

We know of no commercial pilot currently flying whose migraines are likely to interfere with the safe handling of his aircraft.

Cold: Prolonged exposure to cold has frequently been reported as a migraine trigger; however, little research has been done in this area. Some find that the effects of cold are aggravated by wind.

Heat: Many find that they cannot stretch out on a beach chair and bask in the sun without feeling the first twinges of an oncoming migraine attack. The problem is intensified when heat is accompanied by high humidity. (This is the type of weather that often breeds thunderstorms, which are preceded and accompanied by low barometric pressure.)

Women (and men, too) often complain that they cannot tolerate the heat of hair dryers used in salons. (Curlers used in applying permanent waves, and even the massage applied during the washing of hair in a salon are other frequently-reported problems.)

Wind: Some sufferers find that whenever their head is exposed to strong wind over long periods of time a migraine will develop. By far the most serious problems are caused by the famous hot, dry winds of the world, including the sharav of Israel, the Santa Ana of southern California, the Arizona desert winds, the zonda of Argentina, the Mediterranean sirocco, the Maltese Xlokk, the chamsin of the Arab countries, the north winds of Melbourne and the foehn of Switzerland, southern Germany and Austria. (The winter chinook of Alberta and France's mistral are classified as cool winds, though the chinook can raise temperatures in its path by forty degrees fahrenheit in a mere quarter of an hour.) These hot winds can be counted upon to spark an epidemic of migraine attacks whenever they appear. And they may well have other effects on health both physical and mental—stories of strange and unaccountable human behavior are legion.

Professor Felix Sulman has studied these hot winds and their strange effects, and believes that the weather front routinely preceding the winds' arrival and bearing increased ionization of the air (electrical charges often responsible for lightning) may be responsible for the migraine symptoms.

The question of ions and their role in weather-related health disturbances including migraine remains controversial. There is no doubt that the atmosphere becomes infused with positively charged ions prior to a storm and that the storm itself releases negative ions which again neutralize the atmosphere. Some research has indicated that the temporary surplus of positive ions is responsible for the problems experienced by weather-sensitive people and that they could be helped by exposure to air containing negatively-charged ions. To this end, a number of companies have begun manufacturing negative ion generators of various degrees of size and complexity. However there is still no conclusive evidence that they do indeed help to relieve weather-borne symptoms in migraine sufferers.

FOODS, DRUGS AND MIGRAINE

Although the link between migraine attacks and various foods and drinks has been known, or at least suspected, for several centuries, the first serious research into the subject was under-taken just a decade ago, by Dr. Edda Hanington, herself a sufferer. Her work concentrated on two amines contained in foods frequently reported to have the ability to trigger migraine attacks: tyramine (found in cheeses) and beta-phenylethylamine (found in chocolate). Her tests seemed to show conclusively that these amines had the ability to trigger migraine attacks in sufferers. But the experiments were not duplicated and con-firmed, and, over the years, a degree of skepticism about her results began creeping into the study of migraine. This, despite the overwhelming weight of anecdotal evidence supplied by migraine sufferers themselves, few of whom have ever had any doubt about the link between some kinds of foods and their attacks. An elaborate study of migraine and food done in Britain by the National Hospital for Nervous Diseases and the Department of Immunology, Middlesex Hospital, gave the connection added interest. This should open the way for further examination of specific foodstuffs to try to determine the exact chemical nature of their triggering mechanisms. The foods involved in this most recent study were: milk, tea, oranges, apples, cheese, tomatoes, fish, eggs, coffee, wheat, chocolate, shellfish and rice.

Dr. Hanington surveyed five hundred dietary migraine sufferers, and they reported the following foods as triggers in order of frequency:

Chocolate   75%
Cheese and dairy products   48%
Citrus fruits   30%
Alcoholic drinks   25%
Fatty fried food   18%
Vegetables (especially onions)   18%
Tea and coffee   14%
Meat (especially pork)   14%
Seafood   10%

Our own list (which follows) is somewhat more extensive, compiled as it is from the results of contacts with thousands of sufferers. In most cases, there has been no scientific testing done to confirm these reports; however, we have been careful to include only those food triggers which have been reported frequently enough to satisfy us that there is indeed a linkage between them and migraine attacks in some sufferers. Remember that not all migraine sufferers are affected by all of the foods listed: in fact, some sufferers are not affected at all by foods. Most will find that only two or three or perhaps a few more must be avoided (and avoided completely: don't forget about licking spoons or testing during preparation even though you may not eat it during the meal).

So don't arbitrarily give up a food because it is on the list, or because your neighbor did and it helped him, or because you had it once and a migraine followed (something else could have triggered the attack), or because you are ready to grasp at any straw which might ease your headaches. Give it up only if you have good reason to suspect it may be causing a problem for you. If an improvement follows, fine. If there is no change, reintroduce it into your diet and move on to the next suspect. And remember that foods you were able to tolerate as a child may act as triggers in your adult body. By the same token, as you move into your fifth and sixth decades, you may find that you are once again able to tolerate foods that were taboo in earlier life. There are no hard and fast rules when it comes to dietary migraine.

Meal Patterns: If cardinal rule number one for migraine sufferers is, "Never sleep in for more than an hour," rule number two must be, "Never go longer than five hours without eating during the day, and never go more than twelve hours between the last meal or snack of the day and breakfast." Going too long without eating can lower the blood sugar content to a point where a migraine can be triggered. Many sufferers report that they must watch their intake of liquids as well—dehydration can bring on a migraine.

Chocolate in any form: This includes candy, sauces, puddings, ice cream, icing, cola soft drinks. Often, chocolate consumed in the form of a dessert or a coated after-dinner mint will not cause as rapid a reaction as when it is consumed on an empty stomach, as a snack. Try carob as a substitute. It tastes very much like chocolate when used in cooking and baking, contains no beta-phenyl-ethylamine and has the added bonus of requiring less sweetening than chocolate. It is low in fat, rich in protein, calcium and potassium and contains small amounts of sodium and iron. It comes in various qualities, so don't give up if the first you try leaves an aftertaste or is in some other way unsatisfactory. Carob can be purchased at most health food stores and is turning up more and more frequently in commercial baked goods.†

---

†One family-owned company is now making and marketing non-additive carob chip cookies nationally. For data contact Dare Cookies, Kitchener, Ontario, Canada. At several points in the text we identify commercial enterprises or products. These are in no way to be understood as commercial endorsements. We do this primarily as a service to migraine sufferers who, we feel, can use as much information with respect to medication and other aids as we can give them.

Cheese and dairy products—especially aged cheese: The older the cheese, in general, the more likely it is to cause a problem. Stilton, aged Canadian and American Cheddar, Brie and Camembert all contain relatively large amounts of tyramine, a known migraine trigger. There is no reason to avoid all cheeses; simply stay away from the mature varieties and cautiously test out others to see which can be tolerated. Watch out for cheeses in sauces, and remember that while a given cheese may not trigger a migraine on its own, it may tip the balance when consumed along with other triggers like red wine.

Yogurt, sour cream and cottage cheese are the dairy products mentioned most frequently after cheese. Lower down on the list come powdered milk and heavy cream and, last of all, ordinary milk. (Watch out for the synthetic coffee "creamers" or "whiteners" used as substitutes for cream: they too can sometimes trigger attacks.)

Citrus fruits: Some report that they must eschew them all: oranges, lemons, limes, grapefruit. Others say that only oranges cause a problem. Citrus peel in fruitcake may or may not be tolerated.

Bananas: These are a problem for many, either eaten raw, or cooked in banana cakes and loafs. One of our correspondents reports that he can (and often does) eat them when they are ripe to the point of blackness but that he cannot touch them before that stage. Migraine sufferers in Jamaica have told us they can eat bananas allowed to ripen on the tree. (Outside of the tropics, bananas are of the "shelf-ripened" variety.)

Plums: A small number report that plums cannot be tolerated in any form: ripe or green, fresh or preserved. Many of these same people also find that prunes are a problem.

Apples: This one is really confusing. Some people report that they cannot tolerate apple juice. From Britain, there are reports that unripe green apples are suspect. In Canada, there have been reports that the kind of apple may be significant: the McIntosh variety grown in eastern Canada may cause problems, while west coast varieties may not. One woman who moved to Canada from the UK reported she had been able to eat apples from Britain, but not those grown in her new home. To further add to the confusion, one man reports he can eat raw apples but cannot tolerate them if they are baked. Clearly, the apple question remains unsettled.

Pineapple: For some, pineapple in all its forms must be avoided. Others are able to tolerate the raw fruit but must avoid it when it is canned in syrup. Still others are affected by pineapple flavoring concentrate. Another unsettled question.

Dried fruit: A small number report they are unable to tolerate any dried fruits. There is no indication whether this applies only to fruits dried with sulphur dioxide (as many are) or to those dried naturally as well.

Fatty fried foods: These are indigestible for many migraine sufferers and seem to trigger an attack by their effect on the stomach and intestines. Among meats, pork is most frequently mentioned, although it is often tolerated when roasted or broiled. Bacon, even when not cured with sodium nitrite, can be a problem when fried. Fried onions have also been reported; but, since onions in any form are often implicated, it is not clear whether the frying process is involved.

Vegetables: Onions and tomatoes head the list. Again, there are variations: some avoid raw tomatoes only, some cannot tolerate them in any form. The same is true of onions. We have heard from one sufferer for whom the mere smell of onions was enough to trigger an attack.

Spinach is mentioned less frequently. It is not clear whether raw spinach has the same effect as the cooked product. Beans of all sorts are also reported to be triggers: broad beans, lima beans, navy beans, green and yellow beans and peanuts (which are also a bean). Some can eat one type and not another; others cannot eat any of them. Some can eat them raw, but not cooked.

Tea and coffee: Many sufferers reach for black tea or coffee at the onset of a migraine to help constrict the blood vessels. Indeed, there are those who are able to control their attacks simply by taking caffeine in the form of tea or coffee together with an over-the-counter analgesic or a small dose of ergotamine. On the other hand, many who enjoy (or feel they need) relatively large amounts of tea or coffee during the day find that this can trigger an attack, or at least act as a contributing factor. If caffeine is withdrawn suddenly, a blockbuster migraine can result (perhaps due to the rebound effect on vessels long-constricted by caffeine).

Decaffeinated coffee is used by a great many migraine sufferers. (We know of some who keep it around for regular use and have some regular coffee set aside for use when an attack is on the way.) Recently, decaffeinated tea has also become available. In many cases, even the decaffeinated varieties of tea and coffee seem capable of triggering attacks. This would seem to indicate that some factor other than caffeine is involved.

A check of a good health food store will reveal a number of quite acceptable coffee and tea substitutes for those who suspect these beverages may be contributing to their attacks.

Eggs: These are mentioned frequently, but often in connection with bacon or sausage or ham (all of which contain sodium nitrite) and often when fried, so that it is not clear whether the eggs themselves are causing the problem. However, we have also received reports from those who cannot tolerate eggs that have been boiled, shirred or baked or used in soufflés or custards or quiches. A very few people have reported being unable to tolerate egg whites alone.

Seafood and fish: Seafood is by far the great problem. Although it may be just wishful thinking, some report that they can tolerate it in small amounts, as in a shrimp salad or lobster bisque.

Fish is reported less frequently, and then often in the context of fish and chips, where it is not then clear whether the fish itself or the frying process is operative. Sardines and herring are also sometimes reported; however, both come preserved in a bewildering number of ways, and it is difficult to know whether the problem lies in the fish or in the canning methods.

Nuts: First on the list are peanuts and peanut butter (yes, yes, it is really a bean!), then walnuts, pecans and almonds. Farther down the list are coconut, cashews, pistachios and all other nuts. For many, the chocolate-and-nut or dried fruit-and-nut combinations are double trouble. Some find that salted nuts are more likely to trigger an attack than those which are dry roasted.

And let us not forget the avocado "pear," which is really a nut. We know of one man who travelled from Britain to California once every three years to spend some time with his in-laws. Each visit would be marked by an almost continuous migraine. His in-laws own and live on a large avocado farm and employ a Mexican cook who knows scores of ways to prepare avocado dishes, at least one of which was served virtually every day. Now the man continues his regular visits, but the cook is asked to put aside her avocado repertoire for the duration of his stay.

Wheat: Many migraine sufferers cannot handle wheat in any form and must live according to the DEAMOF rule (Don't Eat Anything Made of Flour). It is not unusual to find immigrants to North America who were able to eat pasta and bread in their homeland but who cannot tolerate products made from the hard varieties of wheat grown in North America.

We have the public health nurses of the Canadian Prairies to thank for uncovering one bread-related migraine trigger. Most cookbooks produced in North America are written and tested in the low-lying areas of the eastern and western seaboards or near the Great Lakes, where the major cultural centers are located. Many cooks on the Canadian Prairies and in the plateaus of the American Midwest have failed to recognize that anything made with yeast according to recipes found in these books will not rise properly in the time allotted, because of the difference in altitude. If breads or rolls baked without adequate rising time are eaten within twenty-four hours of leaving the oven, they can cause a "raw yeast" migraine. A good rule of thumb for high-altitude books is to increase the rising time allowed in most cookbooks by 25 or 30%.

Licorice: Licorice in any form, including anise-based liqueurs such as anisette.

The Hot Dog headache: Some sufferers develop an attack shortly after eating hot dogs, bacon, ham, salami or other cured meats. The culprit is a food additive called sodium nitrite, which is a vaso-active agent: it causes blood vessels to dilate. Nitrites are added to the salt used in the curing process to give the meats a uniform red color. Without them, impurities in the salt can leave the meat looking splotchy. Nitrites in bacon or sausage are often a contributing factor in weekend migraines, via the traditional pancake-and-sausage or bacon-and-egg Sunday breakfast. The amount of sodium nitrite in a given piece of meat can be reduced by leaving it unwrapped and unrefrigerated for a time: an hour at room temperature will generally affect a 10% reduction in nitrite content. This, unfortunately, does not work with hot dogs and sausages encased in their own wrappings.

The Chinese restaurant syndrome: Another common food additive which causes blood vessels to dilate and which can thereby trigger migraine attacks is monosodium glutamate, better known as MSG. It is used to excess most often in Chinese restaurants, where it is valued for the bright coloration it gives to vegetables and sauces. It is also considered to be a flavor enhancer. You don't have to be susceptible to migraine to suffer the effects of MSG; but it helps. The usual symptoms are a sensation of pressure or tightness in the face, a burning sensation over the neck, shoulders and torso and a painful pressing feeling in the chest. Some victims complain of mental confusion, disorientation and blurred vision. All of this may be accompanied by a severe headache, especially in victims of migraine. In a few cases, the symptoms have become so severe that a victim has lost consciousness or been admitted to hospital for observation.

The symptoms may persist long after the meal has been consumed.

The effects of MSG on the body are most pronounced when it is consumed on an empty stomach. In many Chinese restaurants the won ton soup served prior to the main course is liberally laced with MSG: one test found three grams per seven-ounce serving. So if you don't want to give up on your favorite Chinese restaurant, make sure you eat a roll or something else before getting into the won ton. (Of course, not all Chinese restaurants use MSG. Any first-rate chef frowns upon the stuff, since, if fresh produce is carefully prepared, no flavor or color enhancer is necessary.)

MSG is also found in a variety of canned, dried, packaged and frozen foods. It is found as well in some prepared meat seasonings. One of our correspondents reports having had a migraine attack at about ten o'clock most summer evenings. He enjoyed barbecuing steaks, and habitually seasoned them with a concoction which contained MSG. The headaches followed each meal by about thirty minutes—until he switched seasonings.

The Ice Cream headache: Many people, whether migraine sufferers or not, have experienced the piercing head pain that can result from eating very cold ice cream. Occasionally, this pain can trigger a migraine in sensitive subjects. The problem is not the ice cream itself, but its coldness. The sudden cooling of the roof of the mouth affects nerve endings which refer pain to the temples and forehead. There is no truth to the old wives' tales that the ice cream headache results from the ice cream (or any other ice-cold food) "hitting the stomach," or that a headache will result from eating an ice cream dessert following a fish dinner.

Writer James Jones, in a short story, suggests that the ice cream headache may have some educational value. Writing of the relationship between a grandfather and his grandchildren, he says: "He loved to feed them large doses of ice cream on summer afternoons, would laugh at them gently when they got the terrible sharp headaches from eating too much too fast, and then give them a gentle lecture on gluttony."

Fever: The fever that accompanies a cold, flu, grippe or myriad of childhood diseases, can be the cause of a migraine attack. When this happens, be certain to contact your physician before using a vaso-constricting migraine medication such as ergotamine. Such drugs can sometimes be dangerous when used in the presence of a high or continuing fever.

Rebound migraine: The habitual use of such vascular-constricting agents as caffeine in tea, coffee and some over-the-counter analgesics, nicotine in tobacco and migraine medications such as ergotamine, can lead to a rebound or withdrawal migraine when their use is abruptly discontinued. The blood vessels have been kept in a continuous state of relative constriction, and when the constricting agent is removed, they rebound to their normal state, causing a headache. This is part of the reason why migraine sufferers are strongly advised against taking ergotamine medications on a daily basis as a preventive. In preventing one attack, they are simply laying the groundwork for another. It is not unusual for sufferers who have overused ergotamine to require hospitalization (and perhaps to be "covered" with other medication) as the use of ergot is withdrawn.

Anesthetics: General anesthetics used in surgery can cause problems in two ways: the anesthetics themselves can trigger a migraine which will appear on regaining consciousness; the requirement of an empty stomach may mean twelve or more hours of fasting prior to receiving the anesthetic. It is not unusual for someone to be wheeled into the operating room with a low blood-sugar-triggered migraine in progress.

The surgeon should be informed that you are subject to migraines. Once he knows this, he may elect to order intravenous feeding prior to the operation to avoid a migraine attack caused by fasting. He can also see that your migraine medication (if any) is noted on your chart. Ideally, such medication should be on hand at the nurses' station so that it can be administered on short notice, as soon as the first signs of a post-operative migraine develop. Otherwise the attending nurse has to seek a physician's approval to administer the medication, and then it must be ordered from the hospital pharmacy. By the time it has been delivered, the attack may be well under way, in which case the medication will be of little or no benefit.

There may be occasions when migraine medication is contraindicated by the type of surgery that has been performed, but, in general, most surgeons would prefer to see their patients free of migraine so that the body's full resources can be devoted to post-operative recovery.

Sleeping pills: Sleeping pills produce an unnatural sleep which can trigger a migraine attack. Relaxation techniques and other more natural methods of inducing sleep are to be preferred.

Allergies: Many season migraines—those which occur regularly in the spring or in late summer or early autumn—seem to be related to histamine-producing agents in the air. The migraine sufferer may have a mild reaction to spores, pollen or other agents, perhaps not sufficient to be classified as an "allergic" reaction, but sufficient to cause the body to produce enough histamine to worsen an existing migraine or to combine with other triggers to provoke an attack.

Migraine victims can have allergies, just like anybody else, and an allergic reaction can trigger a migraine attack. One young woman we know of came to expect a migraine every time she visited certain relatives and, at the suggestion of well-meaning friends, spent a lot of time searching within herself for some hidden resentment or dislike. However it was not her relatives but their cats that were at the root of the problem; the woman was allergic to cats, and being near them brought on puffy eyes, a runny nose and a migraine attack.

It is not uncommon for there to be some diagnostic confusion between migraine and allergies, since migraine can sometimes closely mimic the symptoms of a strong allergic reaction. Many migraine sufferers will awaken in the morning with all the usual symptoms of a migraine attack, plus a runny nose or sniffles, or a blocked nostril. The migraine pain may be located in the cheeks and sinus area around and above the nose. (This can also lead to a mistaken diagnosis of "sinus problems," acute infection, and rhinitis. Fortunately, tests for these conditions are straightforward, and the results are seldom equivocal.)

However, if you suspect you may have allergies in addition to migraine, you should discuss the matter with your family physician to see if a referral to an allergist for testing should be considered.

A word of caution: a migraine attack can raise the histamine level in the blood, just as an allergic reaction does. If, when the allergy tests are done, you are experiencing an attack, or about to have one, or if you have had one within the past day and a half, the results of the test *could* be invalid, and re-testing during a migraine-free period would be required. We have seen a number of people go through all of the inconvenience of weekly allergy shots to no avail because their problem was actually migraine.

(Incidentally, no matter how closely a migraine attack mimics an allergic reaction, antihistamines do nothing to alleviate the problem. Logically they should; but they don't. Sometimes the aspirin or other analgesic usually combined with antihistamine in non-prescription medications will be of some help, particularly if the stuff is taken very early on in an attack, and the benefits may then be wrongly ascribed to the antihistamine.)

Nitroglycerin: It has long been known that people who work in plants where nitroglycerin is made or used are often subject to severe vascular headaches. The effect is compounded in migraine subjects. Once again, it is the nitrite which, as a vaso-active agent, causes the problem by dilating the blood vessels. Alfred Nobel, who worked with nitroglycerin in inventing dynamite, suffered from severe migraine attacks.

People who suffer from angina pectoris (a constricting of blood vessels affecting the functioning of important heart muscles) are often supplied by their doctors with nitroglycerin tablets to be dissolved under the tongue when an attack occurs. Some report a quick, often searing headache following use of the pills. This can cause a problem if the angina sufferer is also prone to migraines, and it may call for some joint consultation between the patient's neurologist and cardiologist. Keep in mind that, on rare occasions, a severe migraine attack can mimic some of the symptoms of angina (See Chapter 2).

Alcohol: An incident from my own naïve youth comes to mind: I recall, too vividly, having a prize hangover (or so I thought) the morning after having consumed just two glasses of red wine. Wondering aloud how this could be so, I was met with ill-concealed skepticism from friends and colleagues who quite logically doubted my protestations of moderation. " 'Two glasses,' you say. Really!" I now know that the "hangover" was actually a first-class migraine.

Later on in life (and still naïve) I, for a time, made a practice of enjoying a lady-like glass of sherry as an aperitif during my lunch breaks. On returning to work, I would suffer through the afternoon with a migraine headache, which I attributed to stale air, the tedium of work, to just about everything but the glass of sherry. But it was the sherry that did it.

There are still some migraine sufferers who are not aware that alcohol, in any form, dilates the blood vessels and can thus trigger a migraine attack or severely aggravate an attack already in progress. While alcohol in moderation can sometimes ease a tension headache, it can only make matters worse where migraine is concerned. Going into a migraine, during the attack itself and usually the day after as well, alcohol in all its forms should be strictly avoided.

In addition to being a potent dilator of blood vessels in itself, alcohol in some forms, notably red wines, contains both tyramine and histamine, both of which are equally vaso-active agents capable of enlarging blood vessels.

We suggest that migraine sufferers consider only those alcoholic drinks that have been highly distilled. Easier still—follow the rule of thumb which suggests avoiding any alcohol that is colored. This leaves vodka, gin and white wine as the most common possibilities for indulging yourself when you are migraine-free, without bringing on a headache.

With respect to beer, some tell us they can handle it in the winter but not on a hot summer day; others tell us that European beer does not produce as many migraines as can the beers made in North America. Still others claim that they can drink only specific brands. We think the beer and ale question is far from settled.

When wine or other alcohols are used in cooking, the alcohol itself is generally completely gone through evaporation by the time the food is ready to serve; however, any histamine content will remain in the food. So it often pays to be wary of those sauces and desserts which call for such things as wine or brandy in their preparation if you are among those who are quite sensitive to histamine.

While on the subject of alcohol, we may as well point out that hangover headaches are vascular in nature just like migraines, though the pain is seldom as intense as even milder migraine attacks. Coffee will do nothing to sober you up, though it may produce a hyperactive drunk. The morning after, coffee and tea can help, since caffeine acts to constrict blood vessels which have been painfully enlarged by the alcohol in the system.

General Ulysses S. Grant suffered from migraine and used to regularly drink himself into oblivion to escape the pain. He would routinely awaken the next morning with both a migraine and a hangover headache. He did, however, discover a once-in-a-lifetime cure: his diary notes that on the morning of Appomattox, he felt unspeakably wretched until the news of Lee's willingness to surrender was delivered to him, whereupon, he says, his migraine eased instantly. He never did learn that alcohol can only aggravate migraine.

CHAPTER 5

Some Tips
for
Self-help

Once migraine triggers have been isolated, it will often be found that avoidance is the simplest and most obvious form of self-help. In other cases, the answer will not be quite so straightforward. What follows is a series of tips for self-help which are the direct result of years of experience working with migraine sufferers and medical specialists.

If you suffer from migraines, you deserve the sympathy and understanding of those around you. And you can help them to understand by providing them with information about your condition. You might arrange a joint consultation with your physician so that your wife or husband can find out about the condition from an authoritative source (assuming that your physician is indeed an authoritative source of information on migraine). Or you may wish to write to one of the agencies or foundations listed at the back of this book; they will provide papers and pamphlets on migraine free of charge. These agencies and foundations can also be of help if you have a specific problem at work or school which needs the understanding and co-operation of someone in authority for its solution.

Parents of small children have a special problem: children

need constant attention, and, until they reach a certain age, it is difficult, if not impossible, to get them to understand that a parent who is suffering a migraine attack needs peace and quiet. If baby-sitting can be arranged reliably on short notice, perhaps through a swap arrangement with another migraine parent, you can get them out of your hair while you try to cope with your migraine. An understanding spouse can also be a big help by keeping the children occupied quietly; unfortunately, he or she may not always be available when you need help most. We found a deceptively simple way to convey to children the idea that mother is hurting and needs to be left along as much as possible: when you feel a migraine coming on, put a Band-aid on your forehead. The children identify the Band-aid with pain and injury and are extra-considerate. Try it: it works.

EXERCISE AND RELAXATION

Keeping the vascular system toned up is, perhaps, even more important in migraine sufferers than it is in the rest of the population, and the same can be said of developing the ability to relax. In some ways, the two go hand in hand, since the right kind of exercise can be an excellent aid to relaxation. One specialist, Dr. Arnold Friedman, has characterized the benefits of a program of moderate exercise as "striking." But it is important to choose the form of exercise carefully.

Those whose attacks are mild and infrequent can often participate in such sports as downhill skiing, tennis, swimming and jogging without ill effects. It is a wise precaution, however, to speak with your doctor before undertaking any of the more strenuous sports—particularly if you are taking migraine medication.

Remember to start off gradually. Easy does it is a good rule. If, in the first day or so, you find that a migraine problem is cropping up in connection with the activity, stop. Try something else. You may later be able to go back to the original activity, once your body is better conditioned to accept it.

Very generally speaking, for those adults who suffer severe migraine attacks, the consensus seems to be:

Tennis: No—and "no" to being a spectator.

Golf: Yes—provided glare-proof sun glasses are worn.

Jogging: This very fashionable form of exercise is capable of causing instant migraines among many sufferers. Some find the attack comes immediately upon returning home; others experience an attack within the first few blocks of running. A few have lost consciousness while jogging. Nevertheless, some *men* report benefits.

Walking: Yes! This seems to be the best form of exercise for us. In good weather, try to plan a daily walk. But don't set yourself unreasonable goals; work up to it gradually, and avoid the guilt associated with unfulfilled goals.

If you are considering regular attendance at a supervised class or club, or at a commercial "spa" operation, speak to the instructors before signing up. You will need to know the kinds of exercise involved (whether, for example, any of them require a head-down bending or stooping attitude), how quickly the program increases the degree of difficulty of the exercises and whether or not the program is flexible enough to include alternatives to activities which may trigger migraines.

Try to arrange a trial use of the facilities, to avoid later problems with refunds on fees paid in advance. Once their money has been invested, too many sufferers try to continue with an exercise program even though it may trigger attacks, or they may insist on attending on the day after an attack. Either can be dangerous. While a few find that exercise seems to aid in recovery from migraine hangover (that feeling the day after an attack, when you are no longer afraid of living but hope someone got the licence number of the truck that hit you), most find that exercise too soon after an attack will only bring on another.

If a contract is involved in your exercise scheme, add a

clause stating that it may be cancelled (with an appropriate refund) if the program becomes too taxing. Remember that both parties to the contract must initial the clause. Without this precaution, you could join those we know of who have lost hundreds of dollars by joining programs they were unable to tolerate.

Gardening is a gentle pastime, providing both exercise and relaxation. But try to avoid stooping or bending. Use long-handled tools where possible, or arrange your garden so that you can sit on a mat and work with the plants somewhere close to eye-level. Take it easy at the beginning: stiff and sore shoulders, backs and necks can lead to aching heads. Wear a loose-fitting cap or bonnet and plan your work for the morning or evening when the sun is not at peak intensity.

Many household chores provide beneficial exercise if care is taken to avoid triggering an attack. Don't over-exert yourself and try, once again, to arrange work so as to avoid bending and stooping. Mowing the lawn is obviously done walking erect, but watch out for the dandelion digging and edge trimming. Long-handled tools are available to do these jobs.

Shovelling snow severely aggravates more migraine attacks than probably any other job around the house. It can be extremely heavy work, particularly when the snow is wet. You might be better off to hire the neighbor's boy or girl to do the job, or buy a snow blower.

If you find that you must lift heavy objects, do it correctly: bend the knees; grasp the object; keep the back straight and the head erect, and lift using the leg muscles.

Relaxation techniques can do wonders in alleviating migraine problems, particularly when the attacks are triggered by tension headaches. (Some of the more effective techniques are dealt with in detail in Chapter 7.) Dr. Arnold Friedman recommends seeking out "a knowledgeable conductor of exercise classes who includes in the regimen movements that are specifically designed to relax taut muscles, or ask the family physician to recommend a physiotherapist who can offer such instructions."

Bad working habits can also contribute to tension head-aches: a typewriter placed so low that it forces you into a crouch; a chair that does not give back support (at work, ask for a model that fits you—it will quickly pay for itself in increased productivity and fewer errors); prolonged reading under poor light and so on. Poor posture, if assumed continuously, will tense muscles and contribute to muscle-contraction headaches. If the posture isn't corrected, shoulder and neck muscles can often become so contracted that the ensuing headache can become almost continuous and severe enough to mimic a migraine. Exercise is the recommended therapy, along with the application of heat by means of hot packs, hot water bottles or heating pads, or, perhaps, a protracted stay under a warm shower. Massage can also be a big help in relaxing tight muscles but it is sometimes difficult to find a skilled professional—the ministrations of an unskilled practitioner can sometimes do more harm than good. Ask your doctor. Massage therapy is suggested for tension headaches both before and during bouts. It will do little or no good during a migraine attack, even if the attack was triggered by a tension headache.

Too much relaxation, in the form of an abrupt come-down from stress, is one of the more common migraine triggers. The so-called weekend migraine, which is more often than not related to too much sleep, is a good example. The solution is simple: never sleep in more than an hour on the weekend. Only if illness is present or if some serious emotional difficulty has been encoun-tered during the week, will more than an extra hour's sleep be necessary to completely revitalize the body. In these cases, it is the experience of most of us that nature lets us get away with sleeping in without adding a migraine to our problems. Some people find this advice difficult to follow, arguing, "I may not need the extra sleep; but I *deserve* it," or, "If it feels so good, it can't be bad." In these cases, a little lateral thinking may be called for. One of my favorite cases involves a man who absolutely refused to give up his habit of sleeping in for as long as was decently possible on Saturdays and Sundays, even though he knew the odds were excellent that this was the cause of his recurring weekend migraines. His wife begged, pleaded and cajoled, to no effect. One day, in a moment of inspiration, she bought him a dog. The man became so fond of the animal that he now quite willingly gets out of bed early in the morning to take the dog for a walk. The frequency of his migraine attacks has dropped dramatically.

Vacation time also produces opportunities for the stress come-down migraine to surface. The problem is often magnified by the extra stress involved in packing and making other travel arrangements during the days preceding departure on a vacation trip. From that, straight into complete and utter relaxation can trigger a blockbuster of a migraine. The trick is to plan in the first few days of the vacation to be up and moderately active relatively early in the mornings and then, over the course of the holiday, to come down slowly and easily.

In other cases an orderly and sedate existence may be the norm, and a vacation may be a time of sudden stimulus involving new sights, unfamiliar foods, increased activity and late nights. In these cases, problems with migraine can be reduced or avoided by rationing change and excitement for the first few days, making the transition between styles of living less abrupt.

We frequently hear from sufferers who have been through periods of intense stress at work or in their family life and who have handled them successfully, only to come down with a severe attack after the fact. They often seem to feel that the fates have been especially unkind to them, that their migraine attack was somehow a low blow. "But I went through the whole time without getting an attack, and then, just when it was all over with . . . ." After this has happened a couple of times, it should be seen, not as a punishment, but as a normal pattern of stress followed by migraine, and then some simple planning can be done to lessen the problem. Find some other engaging activity to follow a time of predictable stress: for the person in this situation, a change is better than a rest. Don't hesitate to discuss your problem with your physician, who may choose to change your medication to get you through the period of stress come-down. Remember, migraine is not an emotional problem that can be willed away. It is a physical condition, and it sometimes requires medication to control it, regardless of one's mental or emotional strengths or weaknesses.

In some cases, stress come-down migraine can be a daily occurrence. One such case reported to us involved a migraine sufferer who had to fight his way home each weekday through rush-hour traffic, the late afternoon sun, often dead ahead, aggravating his problem. His sympathetic wife made a habit of greeting him with a chilled martini after chasing the children out to play, "so Daddy can relax." A short time later, a migraine would develop. It took some coaxing; but the man was eventually persuaded to give up his martini replacing it with a half-hour's meditation on arriving home. Still the migraines persisted—the switch from rush-hour traffic to meditation was too abrupt. In the end, the following plan was developed: after his drive home, he now spends some time in moderately active play with his children, enjoys a quiet family dinner and meditates for half an hour later in the evening. The meditation, he reports, helps him to sleep, and he is better able to handle the drive to work the next morning. The frequency of his migraine attacks has decreased markedly, and it seems safe to assume that his family life has improved in like degree.

SLEEP

As we noted above, too much sleep is a common migraine trigger. Sleep is involved with migraine in other ways as well. It is still the best way to abort an impending attack, and, if it can be managed, it is by far the best way to get through an attack in progress. Frequently, on awakening, the attack will have disappeared.

The amount of sleep required to keep the mind and body functioning at peak capacity varies widely among individuals, but most of us know what our personal requirements are by the time we reach adulthood. Migraine sufferers should try to break their regular sleep patterns as infrequently as possible. Many find that they can get away with one late night; but two or three or more in a row are almost certain to lead to a full-blown attack. This is true of children as well, and their adult guardians have a responsibility to see that they maintain regular sleep patterns whether they are at home or away.

Despite the importance of sleep in alleviating migraine problems, the use of sleeping pills should be avoided, except during exceptional circumstances (as, for instance, following surgery or during a severe emotional crisis). The reason is simple enough: there is a difference between sleep induced by drugs and natural sleep, and, while natural sleep is beneficial, drug-induced sleep usually is not. In fact, there is good reason to suspect that the habitual use of sleeping pills can contribute to an increased incidence of migraine attacks. In this, as in the use of all medication, follow the directions of your physician.

Sometimes, migraine sufferers are awakened from a sound sleep by an attack. This usually occurs in the small hours of the morning, around one or two o'clock, or an our or two before one would normally awake—say, at five or six. Or the migraine may be there when the morning alarm goes off. It is not uncommon to awake feeling fine, only to have an attack set in the moment you bend over to turn on a tub or to collect the morning paper from the doorstep (or from behind some nearby shrubbery).

Research at New York's Montefiore Hospital has shown that migraines which occur during sleep are almost always related to periods of rapid eye movement (REM) sleep, rather than to periods of deep sleep. It is during REM sleep that dreams take place and, it is believed, the day's information backlog is sorted, analysed, interpreted and stored. Dreams are often intertwined with the migraines, some research subjects reporting that they dreamed they were having an attack, only to wake up and find to their distress that they were, indeed, in the midst of one. This research has provided an answer to the question of why the timing of nocturnal migraines is coincidental among so many sufferers: barring outside disturbances, REM phases of sleep occur in all of us at roughly the same times during our sleep periods. Still to be answered is the question as to *why* REM sleep and migraine are connected. What triggers nocturnal migraines?

Some researchers believe the trigger may involve changes in brain chemistry, while others suspect that it may be related to changes in carbon dioxide levels in the blood stream during different sleep phases. No one knows for sure.

MEAL PATTERNS

The rule, as with sleep, is to maintain regular habits. Never go more than five hours between the main meals of the day, and never go longer than twelve hours between the last meal of the day and breakfast the following morning. A light snack before retiring is almost always a good idea (provided it's not Cheddar cheese and crackers or chocolate cake or some other food trigger). Similar advice is given to diabetics, who often get headaches if they go too long without eating and thus allow their blood sugar to fall too low. In fact, if you are one of those whose headaches regularly fall into this pattern, your physician may suspect diabetes and wish to do the appropriate diagnostic tests. Diabetics who also suffer from migraines report they have no trouble distinguishing between a migraine and the type of headache involving low blood sugar and insulin. They also report an instinctive feeling that if they eat as soon as they sense the first migraine symptom, an attack may be averted.

If you know that the time between meals will exceed five hours, make some arrangement to have a snack. Many sufferers make a habit of carrying a few biscuits or crackers with them, just in case. Otherwise, it is not always easy to find an appropriate snack when one is required; too often, candy is all that is easily available. Normal nutritional values make candy an unwise choice, and, for those who react to chocolate or nuts or dried fruit, such a snack may only compound their problem. Granola bars are becoming more widely available; but, while these may satisfy the nutritionist, migraine sufferers should check the list of ingredients for such potential triggers as nuts, coconut, soya and dried fruit.

Your bedtime snack need consist of nothing more elaborate than a small bowl of cereal or a slice of toast: in a substantial number of cases, this is all it has taken to eliminate most morning migraines. In any case, it is such a simple idea that it is worth trying.

In general, fasting is ill-advised, whatever its potential benefits may be for the rest of the population.

Weight-loss diets are another area of potential trouble for migraine subjects. Unless there are overriding medical reasons and you are being supervised by a physician, the rule is not to get involved in diets that promise rapid weight loss. Beyond the potential low blood sugar migraine problems they may cause, they are seldom effective in bringing about a long-term weight reduction, since they do little or nothing to fundamentally alter the bad eating habits that caused the initial weight gain. It seems that the most successful diets are those which provide for a slow but steady weight reduction of perhaps a pound a week.

Dieting has become big business. Clubs, organizations and corporations (which pay excellent dividends to their share-holders) offer widely different approaches to weight loss. Study these programs long and carefully before making a decision about getting involved. If possible, speak to a former member, to see if weight loss has been maintained. All of these organizations provide guidelines for daily food intake: some are flexible, and some insist on no deviation whatever. Some of the foods and beverages suggested may be potential migraine triggers: there should be alternatives to these. In some cases, the daily regimen does not allow for a bedtime snack. Some diet schemes include a program of exercise, and this will have to be checked carefully as well, to determine if it can be tolerated.

In most cases, the best plan is to consult your family physician about your weight problem. He or a nutritionist may wish to recommend or can design a sensible program that will have long-term benefits and will help you to avoid the risk of increasing the incidence of migraine attacks.

All of this is even more important where children are concerned, since rapid weight loss (unless required for overriding medical reasons) is potentially more dangerous than it is in adults. It is best to set a goal that can be reached over the course of a year. We have found that post-Christmas season to pre-

Christmas season is the most logical and workable "year" for such a program.

EYE CARE

Contact lenses are a problem for many migraine sufferers. Often, one or both eyeballs begin to bulge during an attack so that, when the eyes are closed, the eyeballs are pressed tight against the lids. This pushes the contact lens against the eye and can cause irritation. While some who suffer only mild or infrequent attacks can get away with wearing contacts if they remember to take them out as soon as an attack starts, it is a wise precaution to discuss the matter with your ophthalmologist and perhaps your physician, and, if you can, arrange for a trial period before investing money.

Sun glasses are the obvious answer to the problem of sunlight and glare; but they must be of the light-polarizing variety and not simple colored glass or plastic. Keep an extra pair around, for insurance. Since most migraine sufferers are subject to some degree of photophobia even between attacks, those who normally wear glasses often report that the new photo-grey lenses which change their tint automatically according to the ambient light are a comfort worth having.

If you are among the many for whom night driving is a migraine trigger, you might wish to experiment with glasses tinted lightly yellow or pink. They can moderate the impact of oncoming lights, without seriously reducing overall visibility.

LIGHTING

In what seems to be a campaign to banish shadows, many public, institutional and commercial buildings are incredibly over-lighted. With the advent of the energy crisis, increasing attention has been paid to this wasteful and pain-inflicting practice, but change is taking place only slowly. Part of the problem is that, in most political jurisdictions, lighting standards written into building codes, or used by architects and designers as guidelines, have been prepared by the lighting industry, whose attitude has been, quite understandably, "More is better." One office we know of is typical: it contains five banks of fluorescent lights running the length of the rather large, windowless room. Workers have found that they have more than enough light to work by with three of the five banks turned off. They are fortunate to be able to turn off those unneeded lights: until very recently, standard building practice was to install just one light switch per floor in office buildings; the lights were all on, or they were all off. The glare set up by typical high-intensity lighting and the absence of soothing shadowed areas can trigger migraines directly, and it can contribute to tension headaches which can in turn trigger migraine attacks. Saner lighting standards produced by independent organizations are no longer difficult to come by, and a photographic light meter can be used to test light intensity where you work. If your office or working space is typical, you will find it is lighted to the same extreme intensity as a television studio: these days cost-conscious managers can be expected to take this kind of information to heart and do something about it. While they are happily saving money by cutting back on lighting, you and your colleagues will be cutting back on your headaches. One major chain of supermarkets in Canada increased its share of the country's retail food business simply by dimming their lights slightly. Surveys had shown that over-lighting combined with a brilliant red and orange decor had been driving customers away, or forcing them to rush their shopping, buying only what was absolutely necessary before fleeing the hostile environment. Everyone benefited from the change, migraine sufferers more than most. Plastic anti-glare shields can be placed over fluorescent light banks to disperse light more effectively and thereby reduce the required number of fluorescent tubes by 25%. Once again, everyone wins. There is also good evidence that "warm" or full-spectrum fluorescent tubes are more easily tolerated than the more usual "cold" fluorescent lights.

The principal source of glare in a typically over-lighted office environment is, of course, the bright white paper on which just about everything is printed. Here, once again, the need to conserve resources has recently brought about some promising new thinking. More and more, paper companies are finding it advantageous to recycle used paper. They have found, however, that the recycled product does not come out as white as the paper produced from fresh pulp wood, and there is an apparent consumer resistance to anything but the whitest of white papers. To some companies, at least, the time seems right for some public education on the virtues of off-white paper. In fact the scientific evidence to support this idea has been around for a long time and is beyond dispute: the most effective color combinations (in terms of ease of reading and reader retention) for any printed message are blue or black print on soft yellow or cream paper—*not* black on white. The switch to pastel or off-white paper stocks would be another change in which everyone wins: the conservationist, the company and those of us who suffer from migraine and/or tension headaches.

Around the home, you can make life more pleasant for yourself and others by replacing standard light switches with rheostats or dimmers. They are inexpensive and easy to install.

Color television can sometimes cause problems for both children and adults who suffer from migraine. One useful trick is to adjust the contrast and brightness controls to reduce the intensity of the color. Some types of lighting effects, animation and rapid-fire editing styles can cause discomfort, and, if they are sustained for any length of time, they can trigger an attack. Whether the offending effect is found in a commercial, a program "billboard" or station break, or in a scheduled program, it is worthwhile to take the time to write a letter to either the chief executive officer of the sponsoring company, or to the television station, informing them of the problem being created for migraine sufferers. Television stations live by their audience numbers, and no company would knowingly spend large sums of money on a commercial which annoys a substantial percentage of its viewers. In this context, even a single letter can have a surprisingly potent effect. It is unlikely that an offending commercial will be withdrawn immediately—that would simply be too expensive; but if the company can be convinced of the validity of the complaint, it will certainly want to use a different approach in its next campaign.

NOISE AND VIBRATION

During a full-blown attack, noise can be one of the most difficult problems to handle. This is the time when you do not want the person next to you clicking away with knitting needles, or chewing celery: it is a time, one husband has told us, when his wife threw a pillow at him for chewing too loudly on a banana.

Noise is also one of the main reasons why those of us who suffer severe migraine may be reluctant to seek help at a hospital. Hospitals, whether on the wards or in their emergency/ casualty sections, tend to produce a lot of noise, most of it of the shattering metal-on-metal variety. The sound of a metal object dropped on a ceramic-tiled floor can send a migraine sufferer into paroxysms of pain.

If you work in a noisy environment, ear protection is the answer. Ear plugs are inconspicuous and do not place any pressure on the scalp (as earphone-type protection may); but, to be truly effective, they should be custom-fitted rather than purchased off the shelf.

The lives of stenographers, secretaries and bosses can be made significantly more pleasant by the use of plastic noise shields now available for most typewriters.

A quiet air conditioner will allow you to close your windows at home when that is necessary to cut out noise from outside. Heavy curtains will further reduce noise transmission through windows.

Most municipal governments have passed anti-noise by-laws at one time or another. More recent laws tend to be quite strict, particularly where the nighttime hours are concerned. You have every right to insist that they be strictly enforced. Have someone call the police.

If you are bothered by noise from a neighboring apartment, hanging a heavy tapestry on the party wall may help cut down high-frequency sound like laughter and conversation. Low-frequency sound such as that produced by the bass line in music played on your neighbor's stereo, is harder to block out. Raising the speakers off the floor by placing them on an open frame or on a thick pad of a sound-absorbing material like styrofoam will help, as will moving the speakers a foot or two away from nearby walls. Both of these practices, incidentally, will also dramatically improve the linearity of the frequency response of most speaker systems; the speakers will reproduce the recorded sound more accurately. Your neighbors may be more amenable to your suggestions for moving their speakers if you approach them armed with this piece of information.

STEAM

When most people think of steam as a possible migraine trigger, they think of it in large volumes: a steam bath or sauna. But, as we pointed out in the preceding chapter, the steam generated by a large holiday meal cooking on an ordinary kitchen stove can also cause a problem for a migrainous cook. A plan we suggested during a television interview just before Christmas some years ago seems to have met with some success: in one case reported to us by a family physician, it allowed a woman to enjoy the first migraine-free Christmas day of her married life. We simply proposed that the turkey or goose might be cooked a day or two before the actual meal and refrigerated. (Dressing must be removed and stored separately or there is a risk of salmonella.) Many people find that this enhances the flavor of fowl, and hot sauces or gravies can be served at the table. You may wish, instead, to purchase a bird already cooked. In either case, the idea is to avoid repeated bending to peer into a steam-laden oven on a day on which there will undoubtedly be plenty of other potential migraine triggers lurking in ambush. With careful planning, many of the side dishes for a festive meal can be partially pre-cooked so that only a few final minutes are needed just before mealtime. You may also wish to substitute dishes which are served cold or raw: fresh vegetables for canapes, salads and chilled soups.

The back-to-basics movement—growing concern about food additives and chemical soil nutrients along with the rising cost of food—has led to a renewal of interest in preserving one's own foods. With this has come an increasing number of reports of steam-related migraines arising out of all the boiling, blanching, simmering and sterilizing that is part of the process. There are some alternatives. You might make an arrangement with a friend to buy certain foods in bulk; you do the freezing or drying and perhaps the peeling, pitting and other preparation work, and he or she does the steamy part. Or you may wish to forget about canning and get involved in freezing or dehydrating instead. If you can't afford a freezer chest, you may be able to borrow or rent space from a neighbor who has one, or there may be a co-operative in your neighborhood.

MOTION

Many of us worry a lot about being stick-in-the-muds, party-poopers or spoil-sports. The feeling is seldom more acute than on a circus midway when the child who is with you begs to be allowed to ride on the Wild Mouse and you can't let her go because she's too young and needs someone to accompany her, and if it's you, you'll end up with a killer migraine an hour later. You can avoid that kind of mental anguish by inviting a third party along—someone who understands your problem and is willing to take the ride with the child.

TRAVEL

In general, take trips in easy stages that allow you to maintain regular eating and sleeping patterns. Plan ahead to avoid getting into situations where you miss meals or spend extended periods without proper sleep.

Take along an extra pair of sun glasses and, if you require them, prescription glasses (and carry a copy of the prescription for your lenses).

Arrange with your physician to have enough of your medication to see you through. Ask the pharmacist to add "for migraine" on the prescription labels, to avoid potential problems with customs officials. It can also help you to explain your condition in a foreign hospital if you should be forced to seek help at any time. It doesn't hurt to have a "To Whom it May Concern" letter from your physician, confirming your migraine diagnosis. If you have ever been accused of being drunk or on drugs while going through the pre-headache phase of a classic migraine attack, you will recognize the potential value of such a letter.

You can provide yourself with an extra bit of psychological insurance, by contacting one of the agencies listed in the back of this book to see if there is a migraine clinic or specialist near where you will be staying while away. Check also with your pharmacist to see if your particular migraine medication is available in the country of destination and if it is sold under the same brand name.

CRAVINGS

When a migraine is approaching or in full force, I confess that I could seriously consider committing a crime in order to obtain very large bowls full of ice cream—especially chocolate ice cream. Under normal circumstances, I'm not even sure I like it.

Many of us have similar cravings for foods that are likely to prolong or intensify our attacks: the ones reported most often are chocolate in almost any form; ice cream or other foods that are very cold; soft drinks; orange juice; heavily salted foods like pretzels, potato chips and crisps; very sweet foods like candy and pastries.

Our only advice is that you not give in. It's not worth it. You may be able to find more benign alternatives to the desired food—carob instead of chocolate, or a spoonful of honey instead of a candy bar or pastry. (But it never quite matches up to the thought of the real thing, does it?)

If you are responsible for a child with migraine, you will have to exercise some firm control in this matter.

CLOTHING

Although inappropriate clothing is more likely to be an aggravating factor rather than a direct trigger, many with severe migraine have had to learn to avoid such garments as turtleneck sweaters or anything with a high or tight collar. Clothing which is tight about any part of the body can become almost impossible to bear during a migraine attack, as can heavy, clunky, noisy bracelets, necklaces or earrings.

Colors and patterns can be important. Like many others, I have learned that a pinstriped suit is a poor investment. Mine makes my vision blur and raises more or less violent protest from my stomach whenever I put it on. But the real fun comes when I try to iron it—the stripes move as though alive. Other geometric patterns and even large prints are also potential problem-causers.

This seems an appropriate place to insert a plea to those who appear on television—especially newscasters—to avoid wearing pinstriped suits or ties. They often seem to move and change color, so that many migraine sufferers find they must avert their eyes to avoid nausea. The viewer's concentration is lost and so is the news that is being broadcast.

Normally, soft, gentle colors are suggested for the basic wardrobe: blue, green, beige, gray. Vibrant colors are left for the accessories. Many people avoid black or navy blue because these tend to emphasize the ashen color one takes on during an attack.

Some textures, notably corduroy, cannot be comfortably worn during a migraine attack because of the supersensitivity that develops in the sense of touch. The wale of corduroy can be so exaggerated that it feels like hills and valleys and gives you the creeps. Taffeta is another problem material, especially moire with its shifting coloration. Leather can feel stiff and unyielding.

During an attack, and even between attacks, nightclothes and bed "linens" made mostly of cotton are more comfortable than those manufactured of man-made fibres such as nylon. Cotton "breathes" well and is relatively inoffensive to the touch.

DECOR

Where a migraine sufferer has a voice in the decorating of a home or office, soft colors will usually predominate. Informal surveys indicate that most sufferers, adults and children, feel better when surrounded by muted shades of blue and green. Those who study the psychology of color say that these shades promote feelings of peace and healing. Geometric designs in contrasting colors (especially black and white) tend to induce nausea, particularly if they cover large areas. Prolonged exposure may even trigger an attack.

When you are decorating, consider carefully how the colors and patterns will be tolerated during a migraine attack. A shocking pink bathroom with black and white floor tiles can look wonderful when you're feeling well; it can also look like the portals of hell when you arrive there after stumbling, hand to mouth, down the hall from your darkened bedroom.

MENSTRUAL MIGRAINE

The first thing to do here is to make certain that your migraines are indeed being caused by hormonal fluctuations and not by some other trigger that appears coincidentally with your period. Many women, for instance, tend to change their dietary habits as their period begins; others go off food completely, forgetting that fasting can unleash a migraine. Still others report that their cravings for certain potentially troublesome foods increase at this time and that their ability to resist these cravings is diminished. (See "Cravings" in this chapter.) Some are in the habit of using alcohol to ease menstrual cramps.

While true menstrual migraine is more difficult to treat than most varieties, there are steps that can be taken. Because of the regularity of the menstrual cycle, it is possible for many women to predict with a high degree of accuracy when their next hormonal migraine will occur. In these cases, a physician may agree to the use of a vaso-constricting agent before retiring for the night on the eve of the anticipated attack. This is one of the very few cases where ergotamine may be used in advance of the onset of head pain. If menstrual migraine is so severe that it seriously disrupts the life of a woman each month, the family physician or consulting neurologist may suggest a migraine prophylactic or preventative medication, which is taken daily beginning a few days prior to the period. Use of such medication may be extended in cases where menstrual migraine is prolonged for days and is, perhaps, coupled with attacks mid-month at the time of ovulation.

A migraine that persists throughout the entire menstrual period should be treated as a single attack. The vaso-constricting medication used at the first sign of the approaching migraine should not be used each day or on *any* subsequent occasion during that attack. Once the blood vessels have enlarged, ergotamine can do little to bring them back to their original shape; only time can help. However, if you have an attack on the first day of your period and then again on the last day, these are obviously two distinct attacks and can be treated as such.

No migraine attack should be an occasion for heroics. The more you make your eyes work, the more you refuse to rest after taking medication, the greater the odds of the attack growing longer and more severe. This is especially true of menstrual migraine. Go easy on yourself. We don't mean to suggest that you must always take to your bed, but do ease your work load and responsibilities. It is not impossible if you plan ahead; the one redeeming feature of menstrual migraine is that its predictability makes such planning feasible.

Finally, here is a brief cautionary tale from Foundation files, which can be taken for what it's worth: a young woman who had rather severe menstrual cramps had to phone her employers at the start of each period to report that she would be absent for at least one day. Apparently the company made allowance for this, and no comment was ever made. However, she developed menstrual migraine, and when she then called in each month as usual, she indicated that the time off was for migraine. After a few months she was fired, having been told that her migraines were causing too much time off work. None of the representations made to the company by interested parties could budge this decision: time lost for a menstrual period was "acceptable"; the same time lost because of migraine was "not acceptable."

A great deal of research is going on into the causes and potential treatment of hormonal migraine. Investigations are underway into medications that might be used specifically for this problem. Other projects are concentrating on new approaches to hormone therapy. The future does contain a glimmer of hope that some of us may not have to wait for menopause to find a measure of relief.

MARIJUANA

In the early years of this century, Canada's Dr. William Osler suggested the use of marijuana to his migraine patients. More recently, the US Surgeon General's initial report on the use of marijuana acknowledged some medical uses, including the treatment of migraine. We know of a number of sufferers who use the drug regularly, and we also know of physicians who believe that it can help relieve pain and nausea.

HOWEVER: a) Marijuana is illegal; b) there are drugs now legally available which do a better job of treating migraine symptoms (though there were not in Dr. Osler's time). Therefore, there is no need for the use of marijuana in treating migraine, and there are very good legal reasons for its avoidance.

Furthermore, we have heard from a significant number of sufferers who report that marijuana has either triggered a migraine or aggravated an existing one.

FOOD AND FASTING

If you suffer from migraines brought on by fasting and you are a Jew or a Moslem, you may think you have a problem. But you don't. We have it on excellent authority that no recognized religion insists that fasts be kept if there is a medical reason to the contrary. Orthodox Jews will probably need a note from their physician for their rabbi at Yom Kippur. Normally, a dispensation allows the migraine sufferer to skip at least half the fast, so that the five-hours-between-meals rule need not be broken.

During Ramadan, Moslems are not expected to fast if doing so causes medical problems: to do so would be against the true meaning of the Koran. The decision is left to the individual, who is expected to know his or her limitations and to live within them.

What is expected is consideration of others who are observing the fast: eat the food you need in private.

IDENTIFICATION

We occasionally hear from victims of severe migraine who, on seeking help in the form of a shot of pain-killer at the emergency department of a hospital, have been turned away or have been subjected to an embarrassing (and necessary, albeit regrettable) cross-examination about their symptoms. This is because someone in the throes of a very severe attack displays many of the symptoms of a drug addict undergoing withdrawal. Frequently, the victim will visit the hospital late at night—the migraine having built up during the day; pupils are dilated; there may be an overproduction of histamine causing sniffles; there is an aversion to light and noise; memory may be impaired so that it is difficult or impossible to recall one's health insurance number, doctor's name or phone number and so on; speech may be impaired; the hands may shake as they tug at an uncomfortably tight collar. It is difficult to blame a harried emergency department nurse or intern for suspecting that they may be dealing with a drug addict looking for a narcotic "fix," particularly if the hospital is located in an area where drug addiction is a serious problem.

The only way to be sure of avoiding this problem is to carry with you some proof of your diagnosis of migraine. This, unfortunately, is not as straightforward a matter as it may seem. Your physician may hesitate at supplying you with a letter confirming your diagnosis, for any number of very good reasons: he may, for instance, fear that abuse of such a document could lead to a narcotic addiction. Or he may fear possible legal ramifications. If he does supply such a letter, it should be re-dated each three or four months, since some physicians will consider such a document of questionable validity if it is more than a few months old. Generally, the original of the document will be what is required, since photocopies are easily doctored.

Such a letter is made more useful if it contains information from your physician as to which medications have proved most useful in alleviating an acute attack in the past.

If you are able to obtain such a document, you should be aware of its value to a drug addict: you have a responsibility to protect it from loss or theft.

The Migraine Foundation has examined the question of identification at great length, and we have concluded that it ought to be possible to issue plastic cards perhaps bearing the sufferer's photograph and signature which would authoritatively confirm the diagnosis of migraine. The medical and legal problems involved are all soluble; the problem of finding adequate funding has so far prevented the scheme from getting beyond the planning stage.

FAMILY LIFE

Some time ago we received a request for help which we found particularly poignant and which said a great deal about migraine-related problems. A young woman told us that her marriage of two years had been unable to withstand the strains imposed on it by her severe migraines and by the guilt and anger that had built up on both sides of the relationship as a result of her condition. She and her husband had sorrowfully split up. But now, they wanted to give the marriage another chance; her husband had asked her what he could do to help her—to help both of them—to live with her migraine. We suggested to her that she tell him this:

Please, just be there!

Accept, as I have, the fact of a chronic medical condition.

Enjoy, as I do, the days when migraine free; but bear with me if there are factors which I prefer to avoid; as always, in the recess of my mind is the need not to trigger a migraine attack.

If necessary, help me, work with me, to isolate what factors may trigger attacks, and let us make a joint effort to avoid such mechanisms.

Gently remind me if you see me being forgetful, about to do something I shouldn't; but bear with me if sometimes I make a conscious decision to take a chance—and don't say, "I told you so" the next morning—but know that I'll act this way infrequently; but there are times I WANT to forget the need to think about migraine consequences.

Accept with me that there might be times when "I" or "we" will have to miss an engagement, will have to change plans—that we'll have to be flexible.

Don't stand up for me, but stand with me, if faced with the myths and misunderstandings that many people nurture in regard to migraine.

If there are times that I ask you to go on without me, do so, without argument and without guilt.

When an attack starts and you recognize the early symptoms, let me take my medication, retire to a darkened, quiet place, to be alone.

But, BE THERE.

Not sympathy nor empathy nor pity is wanted. What is needed is to KNOW that someone who cares is there, someone who *understands*. That someone will look in occasionally to bring a cup of tea, a cold pack and gentle words of encouragement. That someone is there if the attack is lengthy and severe; someone who'll make a decision as to obtaining additional medical help and take it out of my hands.

But, the best gift you can give is to remove my guilt.

And, if possible, remove or solve those matters that I think "must be seen to."

After an attack, the pain may have gone, but I still may not be thinking straight, so bear with me. Don't pose questions which require a major decision—and let me come around gradually.

Hope with me that the attacks will ease or cease as one grows older.

Seek with me the best of medical care. Be with me and encourage me to keep seeking, to try approved therapies, to do as much for myself as I can so that I feel I have a stake in, a part of, a role to play, in finding at least some of the answers to this problem.

Remember, I'm the same person—with or without a migraine.

One woman simply advised her husband: Don't let my migraines become your headaches.

When faced with serious family problems, do not overlook the help that can be offered by counselling from trained psychologists and psychiatrists. It is dangerous to let these problems continue festering.

Occasionally—very occasionally—we run into someone who has developed the unhealthy technique of using the condition to exercise control over a spouse, or to seek attention, so that migraine literally rules the relationship. Clearly, counselling is needed, along with precise medical care in relieving the symptoms and isolating triggers.

More frequent are the cases where the migraine sufferer is accused of bringing on his or her attacks deliberately: "You always get one of your attacks just when we are about to enjoy ourselves," or "I might have known I couldn't bring people home without you getting an attack," or "Every Saturday when I want to go out, you manage to get one of your attacks."

How much better it would be if the family formed a support team to try to help the sufferer isolate potential trigger mechanisms. Then, if a list of triggers should include stress arising out of a lack of self-confidence when faced with unexpected dinner guests, the family can be a cheering squad, helping to find ways of handling stress, perhaps through some form of supportive therapy. Or if the Saturday headache turns out to be caused by breakfast bacon, the whole family could give it up, at least until the sufferer has lost the taste for it.

It is not migraine that destroys relationships; it is plain old everyday ignorance, intolerance and lack of communication.

SOME SMALL COMFORTS

Cold packs are little marvels. Have two, so that one can be left to cool in the refrigerator while the other is in use. They weigh very little so you can apply them, during an attack, wherever they feel best: on the temples, across the forehead, behind the neck, around your wrists. Take them with you when you travel. Airline flight attendants can cool them for you in the galley refrigerator; in a hotel room, you can cool them by running them under cold water in the bathroom sink, or by dropping them in an ice bucket. (Most people prefer not to freeze them because they then become rigid and uncomfortable.)

There is a reason why cold packs feel so good: cold applied to the large arteries of the scalp and neck will constrict them, reducing the pain. Cold also acts as a local anesthetic in the more conventional sense, simply by slowing down the chemical reactions involved in the pain-producing process.

These same gel packs can be heated in hot (not boiling) water for a few minutes. Some sufferers find relief in using a combination of heat and cold applied to their head, heat on top of the head and cold at the temples. As Dr. James Lance has said, heating the small blood vessels of the scalp causes them to enlarge, and that can allow blood to flow out of the tender large arteries.

Another not-uncommon practice is to use cold packs on the head and a warm pack behind the neck to relax tensed muscles. This can be especially effective where a migraine has been triggered by a tension headache.

Some find it helpful to apply heat to the hands and feet while cold is used on the head. During an attack, the extremities often become cold due to poor circulation, and warmth can help bring back the blood supply, bringing down excess blood from the head.

Instant, disposable cold packs which require no refrigeration are also available internationally. The pack, which is covered in a clothlike paper material, is squeezed to release a chemical which cools it to about thirty degrees Fahrenheit within a few seconds. These can be handy to have around, and you can reuse them a few times by putting them in the refrigerator for a while. Avoid using these with young children, since they will not withstand bites.†

---

†Developers of the instant, disposal pack, Kay Laboratories, also has available for hospitals and clinics, large packs which are also activated by hand pressure, but which cover the entire head. It would be interesting to note if these, as is or with refinements,

About 20% of migraine sufferers seem to want the application of heat alone. It is probably a good idea to keep the warmth away from the major arteries of the head in the temples and forehead. *Gentle* heat should always be used. Beware of electric heating pads and other electric appliances: if you fall asleep with some of these gadgets, they can cause severe burns. Sometimes a hand-held hair dryer can be a handy way to apply heat, especially to the top of the head; but the noise may be bothersome.

Occasionally a warm bath will provide some comfort if taken at the first sign of an attack. As well as relaxing tense muscles, it may also help reduce blood flow to the head.

Many swear by a warm shower followed by a cold shower at the first sign of an oncoming attack.

After a bath or a shower, take time to relax, and let the therapy do its job.

Beds that are adjustable so that the head can be cranked up are very nice but, unfortunately, also very expensive. A foam wedge in a washable cloth slip-cover can do the job almost as well and at a lot less expense.

Finally, it is important to learn to live with your migraine, to accept it and adjust to it. There is absolutely nothing to be gained by struggling on when an attack occurs. We'll give the last word here to the American writer Joan Didion, who has suffered from migraine since early childhood:

> *It comes. . . When I am fighting an open guerilla war with my own life, during weeks of small household confusions, lost laundry, unhappy help, cancelled appointments, on days when the telephone rings too much and I get no work done and the wind is coming up. On days like that my friend comes uninvited.*
>
> *And once it comes, now that I am wise in its ways, I no longer fight it. I lie down and let it happen. At first every small*

---

might be beneficial in an emergency/casualty department for severe migraine attacks. (The cost per unit probably puts them beyond the means of the average household.)

apprehension is magnified, every anxiety a pounding terror. Then the pain comes, and I concentrate only on that. Right there is the usefulness of migraine, there in that imposed yoga, the concentration on the pain. For when the pain recedes, ten or twelve hours later, everything goes with it, all the hidden resentments, all the vain anxieties. The migraine has acted as a circuit breaker, and the fuses have emerged intact. There is a pleasant convalescent euphoria. I open the windows and feel the air, eat gratefully, sleep well. I notice the particular nature of a flower in a glass on the stair landing. I count my blessings.†

CHAPTER 6

Treatment of Migraine by Physicians

When physicians discuss the treatment of migraine, they often break the process down into three phases: explanation and reassurance; the removal of triggers; treatment or prophylaxis by medication. This chapter deals with the third phase.

There is a natural and healthy reluctance among many, perhaps most, people to avoid using drugs unless it is absolutely necessary. With migraine, it is often difficult to see why or when the use of drugs might be "necessary." The condition is never life-threatening, nor do any of the drugs currently available hold out any hope of a cure; all they can do is moderate and control. The condition persists whether or not the drugs are taken. In the end, the purpose of the drugs commonly prescribed is to alleviate or avoid pain. For some people that is not quite reason enough. This is particularly true among those who have no clear understanding of what migraine is: those who have a lingering suspicion that it might in some way be "all in the mind" and that given the will, it can be made to go away. The fact that it has not gone away in the past is, for them, merely an indication of insufficient will power.

This, as we have seen, is a delusion: no amount of will power can get rid of migraine headaches. You cannot will an end to a chemical reaction to which heredity has made you physiologically susceptible. You cannot will an end to migraine any more than a diabetic can will an end to his particular condition. Like diabetes, migraine is a fact of life, something that has to be lived with and to which one must adapt. It's that simple. And it is in this context that the use of medications can sometimes make very good sense.

For many, those who suffer only mild and infrequent attacks, specialized medication is not necessary; frequently, a couple of aspirin taken at the first sign of an attack is all that is necessary to make it through the subsequent few hours without undue discomfort. But for others who suffer more frequent and more severe attacks, migraine can cause serious disruptions in their lives and the lives of those around them. As a result, they may become irritable and withdrawn or they may be overwhelmed by guilt and depression. They may become obsessed with their problem, living in terror of the next, inevitable attack. They may even become dependent upon their pain, relying on it to shield them from the responsibilities and realities of everyday life. Serious emotional and psychological problems can develop.

Thus, the real reason for taking migraine medications is not the mere avoidance of pain (however worthy a goal that may be); it is to allow the sufferer to live a normal, productive and satisfying life, relieved, as much as possible, of the guilt and anxiety so often associated with the condition.

There are other, more pragmatic reasons for using a medication prescribed specifically for migraine. Some sufferers who rely on simple over-the-counter analgesics, like aspirin in its various guises, use these medicines so frequently, and in such quantities that they present a serious threat to health. Migraine medications, when prescribed by a knowledgeable physician who monitors their effects carefully, are far safer, and they have an added advantage in that they are usually highly effective, whereas simple analgesics are only occasionally useful.

There is also some evidence that the migraine condition becomes more and more intractable over the years in cases where it goes untreated. Early diagnosis and treatment may avert a situation where migraine has become so entrenched that it responds only slowly or incompletely to migraine-specific medications prescribed later in life.

In a very small number of sufferers, the narrowing of blood vessels feeding the brain during the aura or pre-headache phase of an untreated attack can lead to transient weakness and numbness, or even loss of consciousness. The weakness can be as pronounced as that experienced following a stroke, and it may continue for some time after the head pain has ended. In some cases blood flow to the brain has been so seriously depleted that permanent brain damage resulting in permanent stroke-like disabilities has occurred.

Further, evidence is growing that year after year of untreated severe migraine can lead to high blood pressure, which, if also left untreated, can cause serious medical problems. Those who refuse treatment may also pay for their obstinacy in later years through impaired hearing and vision.

(We should like to make it clear here, however, that studies comparing the incidence of stroke or vascular accident in migraine sufferers with that of the general population show that they are no more prone to experience stroke than anyone else.)

The point is this: there is no virtue whatever in refusing to use migraine medications if they can help you to lead a happier, more satisfying and productive life. Do discuss it with your physician, or ask him to refer you to a specialist.

MEDICATIONS

Analgesics

Over-the-counter painkillers like aspirin, paracetemol and acetaminophen are sometimes all that is needed to deal with a mild migraine attack; but they are of little or no use in treating a moderate or severe attack. In cases where they do not seem to be effective even in mild attacks, the reason may lie in the fact that they have not been thoroughly absorbed into the system. Aspirin taken in effervescent form is more readily absorbed than the tablets and may be an improvement. Caffeine, either in the form of a cup of coffee or tea, or as an extra ingredient found in some non-prescription painkillers, may also promote more rapid and complete absorption of the aspirin. The key is to take the aspirin or other analgesic as early in the attack as possible, before the pain has become entrenched.

In some cases, a physician may suggest the addition of a small amount of sedative (diazepam or phenobarbital) to these simple analgesics. The rationale for this is that the sedative may help to relieve the pain of an attack by reducing the anxiety associated with it. Since these sedatives can be habit-forming, there is some risk involved here, and it should be discussed carefully with your physician. In general, the routine use of sedatives or tranquilizers in treating migraine is of little or no use. If there is anxiety, it is better treated through explanation of the problem and reassurance that something can be done.

Codeine is available in non-prescription analgesics in some countries, often in combination with aspirin. Used in large enough dosages (30 mg or more) it may be more effective than simple aspirin or acetaminophen. However, codeine is a narcotic, and, if abused, it can become addictive. That is why many countries have removed it from the open shelves in pharmacies. Use codeine-containing compounds only with the advice of a physician, and keep careful track of your consumption.

More potent narcotic painkillers like morphine and meperidine may occasionally be called for to break a very severe attack that has gone on for a long time and got completely out of hand. Administered by injection, these powerful narcotics are dangerously addictive, and they should under no circumstances be used on a regular basis as migraine therapy. (In any case, they are not always effective. See Chapter 3.)

Vaso-constricting Agents

In cases where analgesics are not effective or are effective only in dangerously large dosages, physicians generally turn to an agent which constricts the large blood vessels of the scalp, usually some form or compound of ergotamine tartrate. By reducing the distension of the blood vessels, it reduces or eliminates head pain.

Ergotamine is derived from ergot, a fungus found on the rye plant. Its botanical name is *claviceps purpurea*; it is also known as cockspur rye, hornseed, mother of rye, smut rye and spurred rye. In its raw, natural form it has a foul smell and an unpleasant taste, and it can be quite deadly. In Europe in the fourteenth century ergot began turning up in bread made from rye grain which had been stored too long, and it led to endemic outbreaks of a condition which became known as St. Anthony's Fire. Victims developed a terrible rash, discoloration of the fingers and toes, and, in some cases, entire limbs would putrify and drop from the body, "severed as if by some sudden fire." The only known cure was a pilgrimage to the shrine of St. Anthony in Italy, which, for most northerners, involved a journey of several months' duration. It was an effective cure: as the victims travelled south, the use of rye in bread gave way to the use of other locally-grown grains. By the time the shrine was reached, the body had had a chance to purge itself of ergot, and a complete recovery could be expected. The reason for the dramatic symptoms of St. Anthony's Fire lay in ergot's ability to constrict blood vessels, reducing the flow of blood to such an extent, in some cases, that gangrene developed in the limbs and extremities.

It was not until early in the present century that the ergot derivative, ergotamine tartrate, became available on prescription—the first medication developed specifically for treatment of migraine. In the fifty years since its introduction, other medications have been developed, but ergotamine remains "the Queen of migraine medications," more widely used than any other drug.

Used properly, ergotamine can be extremely effective. *It must be taken at the earliest possible moment, as soon as the first signs of an impending attack are felt.* In classic migraine, this can be when the aura or prodrome first begins to manifest itself. In common migraine it will usually be at the first small sign of pain. Timing is crucial because of the vascular changes which take place during an attack. Following the aura or pre-headache phase, the arteries dilate, and for a brief period, perhaps ten to thirty minutes, dilation is the only abnormality present. Then, kinins and other chemical substances come into play, causing irritation and inflammation of the vessel walls. It is only during the initial ten- to thirty-minute period when dilation alone is present that ergotamine can constrict the vessels. Ergotamine cannot constrict the vessels effectively once the kinins and other substances make their appearance.

In cases where migraine attacks occur with a high degree of predictability—at menstruation, during intercourse, during strenuous physical exercise, in response to a rapid drop in barometric pressure or on long-distance flights—your physician may recommend taking medication even before the first signs of the attack are noticed.

As a rule, however, ergotamine should not be used on a regular basis as a means of warding off attacks. Used daily in this way, it causes more problems than it cures. The blood vessels are kept in a constant state of constriction. When the level of ergotamine in the blood drops between doses, a rebound headache develops as the vessels expand to their normal size. More ergotamine is taken to deal with this rebound headache, and the cycle continues in a downward spiral of head pain of increasing frequency and severity. In such cases of ergotamine dependency, hospitalization may be required so that the drug can be withdrawn under cover of a potent analgesic and/or sedative.

Ergotamine should not be taken where vascular disease (including hypertension) is present. Further, because it is broken down by the liver and excreted by the kidneys, ergotamine should not be used where there is kidney or liver disease, since this may permit the accumulation of toxic levels of the drug even though normal dosages are being used. Finally, because it may present a risk to the developing foetus, ergotamine should not be used during pregnancy, particularly during the first few months.

The most frequent side effects of ergotamine are nausea and vomiting. However, since these are also symptoms of migraine, it can sometimes be difficult to know whether they are a result of the attack or of the drug. Changing the dosage may be the solution.

The effective dosage of ergotamine varies with the individual user, and some experimentation may be necessary to arrive at the best level. So, don't be discouraged if it does not seem to be effective in its initial trials. Talk to your physician and try altering the dosage.

At one time, rather large initial doses of ergotamine were prescribed by physicians—large enough to permit the sufferer to ignore the headache and carry on working. More recently, physicians have tended to prescribe smaller doses and to recommend that the sufferer rest for at least a few minutes after the drug has been taken to give it a chance to begin working.

Ergotamine is available in many different forms, each tailored to suit a specific combination of circumstances. For instance, in pill form it is sometimes combined with caffeine, to promote rapid absorption into the blood stream. It is also available as a rectal suppository and in a form in which it is placed under the tongue to dissolve: both of these methods permit rapid absorption into the blood stream. For those whose headaches are severe and appear without warning, a pressurized nebulizer or inhaler may be the answer: the ergotamine thus inhaled is absorbed quickly and completely by the tiny vessels in the lungs. Physicians treating acute migraine attacks in their offices or in hospital emergency rooms generally elect to use ergotamine by injection, the quickest and most effective method of all.

Remember, ergotamine is potent medicine and must be used carefully. If any unusual symptoms develop, notify your physician immediately.

Sometimes an acute migraine attack will not respond to any of the treatments discussed above and may continue unabated for several days. Sufferers in this condition are usually severely distressed: they may be exhausted, depressed and dehydrated. This extreme condition is known as *status migrainosis,* and hospitalization may be advisable. Rest, sedation and rehydration are important. A quiet, darkened room should be provided, and a major tranquilizer such as chlorpromazine or trifluoperazine may be useful not only for its sedative effect, but also for its anti-vomiting action. In some cases, a narcotic painkiller may be used; but, as we noted earlier, narcotics may be ineffective in combatting the pain of entrenched migraine: their use calls for careful assessment by the physician. Corticosteriods have sometimes been found to be effective in breaking a severe migraine attack; but no one knows why they work. They are generally given by injection as hydrocortisone and prednisolone.

Preventative Medications

In cases where removal of triggers has not reduced the frequency and severity of attacks to an acceptable level, and where treatment with reasonable doses of analgesics or ergotamine compounds has not been effective, a physician may elect to prescribe a migraine prophylactic or preventative to be taken daily. There are a number of such medications, ranging from the mildly effective and quite safe to the very effective and potentially dangerous.

Bellergal is a relatively benign compound described as a "stabilizer of the autonomic nervous system." It contains ergotamine tartrate, belladonna alkaloids and phenobarbital. Side effects are quite uncommon: they can include drowsiness, blurred vision, dry mouth and flushing. It is effective in reducing the frequency of migraine attacks in 30% – 40% of those who try it. Because it is relatively safe and side effects are uncommon, it is sometimes used in treating children, either in the form of ordinary tablets, or in timed-release capsules. Its use is generally withdrawn once the pattern of attacks has been broken. It should not be used by anyone who cannot take ergotamine, or in cases where atropinic substances should not be used (i.e. in the presence of glaucoma).

Pizotyline (Sandomigran) affects the workings of serotonin, histamine and kinins, and this is presumed to be the basis of its effectiveness, which is rated as high as 66% when dosages have been carefully tailored to the sufferer. It may take three or four weeks of steady treatment before its benefits are felt. Side effects are uncommon: they usually consist of drowsiness or heightened appetite, which can lead to an unwanted weight gain. Many users report having unusually vivid and entertaining dreams; few find this a bother. Proper dosage is crucial and can only be arrived at through experimentation, so don't give up on the medication without giving it a fair trial. There are a few contraindications: it should not be used where there is an obstruction between the stomach and the small intestine (pyloro-duodenal obstruction), in cases where the sufferer is taking MAO inhibitors or in the rare cases where a sufferer has a known sensitivity to pizotyline.

Propranolol (Inderol) is one of a family of drugs technically described as "beta receptor blockers." It was developed in the 1960s primarily for use in treating high blood pressure and certain heart problems; but patients using it reported that it alleviated their migraine problems as well. Subsequent research showed that it can be effective in treating migraine in 50% – 60% of cases when used in appropriate dosages and after a reasonable time (four to six weeks) has been allowed for it to begin to work. Why it works is still problematic.

Migraine prophylactics should never be withdrawn suddenly, and this is especially true in the case of propranolol. Not only is there a risk of producing "backlash" or "rebound" headaches, but it may also result in the worsening or "unmasking" of angina pectoris or hyperthyroidism. Withdrawal should take place over a period of at least two weeks. Among side effects are lethargy, upset stomach, a slowing of the heart rate (bradycardia) and low blood pressure. Propranolol should not be used by those with asthma, diabetes, pollen allergies or any history of even mild heart trouble, and it should not be used in the presence of some psychotrophic drugs.

Amitriptyline hydrochloride (Elavil) was originally developed as an anti-depressant; but once again, patients reported that it also seemed to relieve their migraine problems. Subsequent research into its anti-migraine properties showed that it acts on serotonin metabolism. It works just as well with migraine sufferers who have no significant history of depression as with those who do: 50% – 60% of those who use it report it to be an effective migraine preventative. There are side effects; but these can be limited by adjusting the dosage: they include drowsiness, dry mouth, weight gain and constipation. This medication should not be used where heart disease is present.

Methysergide (Sansert) is the original migraine prophylactic, and it remains the most effective. It works in 70% – 80% of cases and frequently works where other agents have failed. It is a derivative of lysergic acid. Despite its relatively long history of use, precisely how it works is still unknown, beyond the fact that it is a serotonin blocker. A response to the drug may be noticed within a few days of beginning its use or it may take up to three weeks for it to take effect. The risk of serious side effects increases the longer the medication is used; it should never be used continuously for longer than six months without discontinuing (slowly) for at least a month. It may then be re-started, provided it is still needed and provided there is no evidence of adverse effects. Some physicians think even six months is too long and interrupt usage every three or four months. If you have been prescribed this drug, you should visit your physician every three months for a blood count, urinalysis, blood pressure and heart and lung check-up. Side effects, though uncommon where the drug is used in proper dosages and for no longer than six months at a time, can be quite serious. Most dangerous, is the development of excess connective tissue in the chest or abdominal cavity (pleural or retroperitoneal fibrosis) affecting lungs, heart, or the kidney drainage ducts (ureters). Less serious side effects are more common and include: nausea, vomiting, heartburn, abdominal discomfort and diarrhea (all of which can be avoided by taking the drug with food); insomnia, excessive dreaming and giddiness (which can be avoided by starting the medication in small doses and increasing them slowly).

A rare side effect may be excessive constriction of the blood vessels, which can lead to serious heart problems. If this is suspected, use of the drug should be discontinued immediately, despite the probability of a rebound headache reaction.

Contraindications to the use of methysergide include heart disease, vascular disease, high blood pressure, phlebitis, fibrotic problems, impaired liver or kidney function and infections and, as with all of the migraine prophylactics, pregnancy.

Because of its potency and the seriousness of potential side effects, methysergide is a medication of last resort, to be used where all others have failed.

Recently, studies of platelet clumping and of prostaglandins (see Chapter 3) and their effects on the development of migraine have led to the use of medications which impede platelet aggregation and interfere with prostoglandins as a means of migraine prevention. These drugs include aspirin, sulphin-pyrazone, tolmetin, indomethacin and others. Early reports were enthusiastic; but later tests indicate that these drugs are not as effective as any of those listed above. The work goes on.

At the present time, there are at least six new medications developed specifically for the treatment of migraine and under-going clinical tests with varying degrees of success. Since it takes years of expensive trials before a new drug can be placed on the market, it will be some time before any of them are available by prescription.

In general, no migraine prophylactic should be used indefi-nitely, no matter how well it works. Use should be carefully tapered off periodically, to determine whether or not the medica-tion is still necessary and to give the system time to "dry out." Often, if a sufferer has been free (or almost free) of headache for several months, he will be able to coast without the drug for a few more months. Many specialists alternate their patients between two different drugs, a few months at a time, to avoid any possible problem with the development of tolerances.

Always remember that migraine prophylactics take time, sometimes several weeks, to begin to do their job effectively. Be patient, and give them a fair trial. There may be times when a particularly bad attack "breaks through" the preventative medi-cation, as when a long period of low barometric pressure piles up the pressures on your system. Any medicine which was capable of averting all of these attacks would truly be a miracle drug. In some cases, it may be permissible to use ergotamine in conjunc-tion with a migraine prophylactic as a means of handling these isolated break-through attacks.

During the past fifty years many different forms of surgery involving both blood vessels and nerves have been used in attempts to alleviate migraine. None has been useful in providing sustained relief. Where one pain pathway has been cut, another usually develops within weeks or months of the operation.

Surgery has fallen even more out of favor with the development of new drugs which treat the condition effectively and at minimal risk to the patient.

Finally, a word about your physician. Assuming that you have succeeded in finding a competent, sympathetic practitioner who makes a point of keeping up to date with the medical literature on migraine, you should be prepared to reciprocate the same trust, patience and forebearance that you expect from him. If the diagnosis of migraine is often tricky, so is effective treatment. The process of finding the right drug in the right combination and the right dosage can be long and frustrating. Follow your physician's instructions exactly, and monitor your symptoms carefully so that you can provide the kind of feedback he needs. If you and your physician can treat your relationship as a sort of creative partnership, your problem will be well on its way to solution.

CHAPTER 7

Alternative Therapies

A number of unorthodox approaches to migraine therapy have, on occasion, given sufferers some relief. When these were reported to the Migraine Foundation, we investigated them as thoroughly as our resources allowed; in some cases we attended training programs established for new practitioners. Our experience leads us to view these forms of therapy as supportive of, rather than alternatives to, standard medical practice as outlined in the preceding chapter. We say this because it has simply been the experience of most of those with whom we have spoken or corresponded that, where these therapies work at all, they generally provide only short-term or limited relief. However there are enough exceptions for whom one or another of these therapies has proved a godsend to make it worthwhile exploring them—with due caution. In medicine, one of the most important warnings for a physician is expressed in the Latin phrase, *primum non nocere,* which can be loosely translated: *at least, do no harm.* Or, to put it another way, the treatment should not be worse than the disease. It is a phrase worth keeping in mind if and when you wish to investigate an approach to migraine therapy that may be outside the current mainstream of medicine.

CLINICAL HYPNOSIS

First, let us discard some misconceptions. Modern medical hypnosis does not involve being put into a deep trance of which you will remember nothing; neither does it involve having the will of the hypnotist imposed on your own. It will not cause you to spontaneously expose the skeletons in the family closet to your therapist nor, for that matter, to do anything else you would not normally do. It is generally a refreshing, stimulating and thoroughly enjoyable experience. It has helped many migraine sufferers to cope with their condition and is often well worthy of investigation. An analogy that comes close to describing the experience is that of talking on the telephone. When you are on the phone you are concentrating on what is being said at the other end of the line; but, at the same time, you are fully aware of everything that is going on around you. If a fire breaks out in your kitchen, you drop the phone.

In general, hypnotherapy is concerned with pragmatic instruction and reinforcement; with the here-and-now rather than with the past. Its goals in treating migraine are threefold: to help the sufferer to avoid triggers (as in the case of dietary triggers and cravings) or to eliminate them (as in the case of psychological stress); to teach the sufferer how to control autonomic systems in the body, in particular the circulatory system. The first two goals are rather obvious; but you may never have thought of the possibilities of the third. It is possible, with proper training and persevering practice, to learn to control the dilation of blood vessels, provided an attack is caught at its very earliest stages. Once dilation is well underway this sort of self-generated therapy is unlikely to be successful. Some people focus on images: one woman we know imagines a sponge wiping away pain and permitting the blood vessels to return to their normal size; another imagines a switchboard and then mentally pulls the plug that carries extra blood to the head. Others simply instruct their blood vessels to return to normal and their hands to grow warm, in order to draw blood down from the head. Relaxation techniques available through self-hypnosis are equally important.

It takes only about half an hour to learn the basics of

self-hypnosis; but follow-up sessions are necessary for learning the techniques of speaking directly to the subconscious and for reinforcement. Mental attitude is all-important and there will be times early on when you will find it difficult to believe that what you are learning to do can actually work. Hence the need for continuing support from the therapist. (The fact is, apart from those who are mentally ill, retarded or brain-damaged, virtually anyone can learn the technique. There is no apparent basis for the belief that some people are "unhypnotizable.") Classes, however, should not go on too long: your goal is self-sufficiency.

Your teacher should be a physician who has had special training in clinical hypnosis. Lay practitioners could involve you in needless risk at worst and waste of time and money at best. Never forget that migraine is an extremely complex medical condition, and its treatment demands specialized knowledge or insight not likely to be found outside the medical profession. (It is rare enough inside the profession.)

Different practitioners employ different techniques in training their patients. We have run across one approach that has caused a problem. Patients were taught to roll their eyes in a certain way to promote increased concentration and the entry into an altered state of consciousness. Rolling the eyes can be a virtual impossibility during an attack; this was clearly not an appropriate form of induction for the migraine sufferer.

Most of those who have trained themselves in self-hypnosis with a physician's help have experienced some degree of relief. Virtually all have found it refreshing, relaxing and interesting, and some have carried on to experiment with its use in other areas of their lives—certainly worth investigation.

BIOFEEDBACK

Another approach to self training involves the use of electronic equipment to monitor and display the workings of the autonomic bodily systems. The monitoring devices provide continuous feedback on the effectiveness of a practitioner's attempts to modify the behavior of a given system and thus serve as a powerful teaching aid. The feedback can be in the form of a changing musical tone, flashing lights, the fluctuations of a meter needle or the scribblings of a stylus on a moving chart. In this way, any number of systems or conditions can be monitored: heart rate, brain waves, temperature, muscle tension, blood pressure and so on. With a little training, it becomes quite a simple matter to control these so-called autonomic bodily functions, through concentration and the use of mental imagery. The precise approach taken to controlling migraine will vary with the individual.

Sometimes a hospital or clinic will have enough equipment to permit trainees to take monitoring devices home for practice. Such devices are also available commercially. An important consideration in the use of such equipment is the type of read-out mechanism employed: a shrill tone or flashing lights may be intolerable during an attack. The ultimate goal, though, is to be able to alter conditions like skin temperature and blood pressure at will without the use of a monitoring device; hence, renting or borrowing the equipment may be preferable to purchasing it.

Generally speaking, a clinic will wish to see you once or twice a week, for a maximum of about twenty sessions. Some people take to the techniques quickly and have the needles dancing at will by the fifth session. Others may require more time. Keep this in mind when you are signing up for a course of instruction: if possible, avoid paying in advance for a set number of lessons because you may not require all of them.

We strongly recommend that you ask your physician's advice in choosing a clinic, since it is important that the technicians be well trained and that the monitoring equipment be well maintained and properly calibrated and, again, that there be an understanding of migraine.

In some countries, biofeedback training, like clinical hypnosis, is covered under medical insurance plans.

If you live in a rural or isolated area and do not have access to clinics, you might want to consider training yourself with the help of a good book on the subject of self-hypnosis or biofeedback. But beware, not all of the books available on these subjects are reliable. Seek the advice of a knowledgeable physician or contact one of the migraine organizations listed in the back of this book.

Once again we stress the need for determining trigger mechanisms as precisely as possible on or before getting involved in biofeedback or any of the other supportive therapies. We know of one man who had an hour's biofeedback training every day after work. At the end of this he felt marvelous; but because the sessions delayed his dinner, he was in the habit of buying a chocolate bar and eating it on the way home. He would crawl into the next day's session with his usual migraine. Until he gave up his chocolate bars, all the biofeedback training in the world wasn't going to help him.

MEDITATION

We are told that transcendental meditation has been of great help to those who suffer from tension headaches, if for no other reason than that the practice involves setting aside some time each day for relaxation and clearing the mind. In those with tension-triggered migraine, a gradual improvement in the ability to handle stress has been reported.

Unlike biofeedback and self-hypnosis, meditation is not generally useful once an attack has begun, since it becomes very difficult to "get in under the pain." Some report that meditating during an attack only serves to make them more keenly aware of their pain, sometimes to such an extent that it floods over them, swamping all other thoughts, emotions and sensations.

Meditation sessions should be scheduled to take place after one has had time to gradually unwind from the stresses of the day: otherwise, they can be a set-up for a stress come-down migraine.

RELAXATION

The sybaritic seventies spawned a plethora of relaxation and stress-relief therapies. Many of these are still around, being taught for a fee by clubs and organizations of various descriptions. Sometimes the instructors are qualified; sometimes they are not. Sometimes the techniques employed are legitimate; sometimes they may be dangerous. Seek advice and proceed with caution.

BEHAVIOR MODIFICATION

Some programs of behavior modification are so dangerous that they have become the subjects of full-blown government inquiries in several jurisdictions. They range from the relatively innocuous and often useful assertiveness training and parent-effectiveness training programs offered by such organizations as the YWCA, to the expensive, obnoxious and potentially damaging "mind development" programs that make fortunes for the moral cretins who run them and leave the landscape littered with emotional cripples. We have heard from far too many people who have had their migraine problems intensified by the bruising techniques employed by some of these programs. We have also heard from many who have been helped by professionally-organized assertiveness-training programs in dealing with the situations behind their stress-related migraine.

YOGA

Yoga encompasses many of the supportive therapies described here. Used properly, it could be better described as a way of life than as a therapy. It requires dedication and instruction from highly qualified teachers; but the rewards are worth the effort involved. We cannot emphasize too strongly that you seek instruction from an expert teacher or yogi who has an understanding of migraine and who can design a program that will ease, rather than aggravate your condition.

ACUPUNCTURE

The technique of acupuncture is based on the knowledge

amassed in *The Yellow Emperor's Classic of Internal Medicine,* said to have been compiled between five and eight thousand years ago in China. In this massive, fifty-eight volume work there is expounded the dualistic philosophy of *yin* and *yang*, from which a system of preventative medicine, including the prevention of pain, is derived.

The ancient Chinese had an approach to dealing with physicians that modern westerners will find thought-provoking. Those who could afford doctors paid them regularly for as long as they (the patients) remained in good health. As soon as illness struck, the doctor's payments stopped, not to be resumed until he had brought the patient back to health. This encouraged the healthy emphasis on preventive medicine which is still the cornerstone of Chinese medical practice.

In this philosophy, illness is said to occur when *ch'i*—life's energy—is out of balance. There are twelve *ch'i* meridians running through the body: six are *yin* and six are *yang*. Together, they represent all of the major bodily organs. Each wrist contains six separate pulses; after a great deal of practice, an acupuncturist/physician can use these in diagnosing imbalances among the *ch'i* meridians. Treatment involves the transfering of *ch'i* from meridians that are strong to those that may be weak, so that balance is maintained in the body's life forces.

The acupuncturist transfers these life forces through the use of acupuncture needles of varying lengths. The needles are extremely fine, finer even than the thinnest of embroidery needles, and their insertion is quick and sure so that almost no pain is felt. Depending on the pulse diagnosis of the patient on the day treatment is to be given, as few as three or four or as many as fifteen or twenty needles may be inserted. They may remain in place for twenty minutes or longer, or they may be twirled in place, at a rate of five twirls per second. Only the wrist of a master acupuncturist with about thirty years' experience can maintain the correct rate of manipulation; in some cases, therefore, a small electric motor is utilized. If any discomfort is experienced, the speed of the motor is adjusted.

You know that you are in the hands of a master acupuncturist if the treatment you receive varies from session to session, based on his diagnosis of your condition on any given day. If treatment is unvarying, it is probably being based on a "recipe book" of acupuncture points.

It is worth keeping in mind that ancient Chinese documents recommend that acupuncture be avoided on wet, rainy days "when the sky is heavy."

In recent years, evidence of acupuncture's effectiveness has gained the technique a measure of respect among western physicians, who now occasionally suggest it as a form of therapy where the condition to be treated is reversible (that is, where organs have not been permanently damaged). Some doctors have even taken short courses in acupuncture and use it in their examining rooms.

If you are considering acupuncture, discuss it with your doctor, and ask for a referral to a *physician* well trained in the technique. Acupuncture should not be used unless there has been a clear diagnosis of migraine, otherwise it may turn off pain that is an urgent warning of a life-threatening condition. Avoid unlicensed backstairs practitioners.

Because of the difficulty in conducting controlled experiments with acupuncture, there has been no scientific validation of the technique's effectiveness in treating migraine. We can only report what we have been told by those who have been in contact with the Foundation. Some have reported receiving dramatic relief. In most cases, however, this has lasted no longer than about three months. Subsequent treatments have not always provided the same level of relief as the first. We have, though, heard from five people in the past six years who have obtained relief for a year or longer.

Some people experienced no change whatever following treatment. In a very small number of cases, patients reported that acupuncture treatment temporarily aggravated their migraine condition. In these cases, their physicians recommended that the treatment be discontinued.

Shiatsu and *an'na* are variations of acupuncture that are generally referred to as acupressure, since the skin is not punctured. Instead, pressure is applied by the fingers, fingernails or needles ending in a ball point. Frequently, when an acupuncturist has located a specific point where stimulation seems to provide help, the patient is instructed in applying acupressure to that point (if he can reach it). There are one or two acupressure points on the body (such as between the thumb and forefinger) that are said to tone up the whole body. The same cautions we applied to acupuncture apply here as well.

MASSAGE

During an attack, a few seconds' relief can often be had by pressing down on the cranial artery on the affected side of the head. You can also frequently get relief by pressing on the carotid artery on the affected side. Obviously, pressure should be maintained for no more than a few seconds, since it is interrupting vital blood supplies to the brain.

Gentle massage of the head and neck may provide some relief where a migraine has been triggered by a tension headache. Used between attacks, more extensive, professional massage can be a relaxing tonic for the whole body. It may be especially useful for those who, for one reason for another, cannot, or do not, exercise regularly. However, during an attack most find even the thought of massage intolerable.

If massage is applied during or immediately following an attack, the masseur should reverse normal practice and work away from, rather than toward, the heart. The leg, for instance, should be worked from the thigh down rather than from the foot up. This is to encourage the flow of blood into the extremities, to warm the hands and feet.

SUBCUTANEOUS STIMULATION

Used widely in pain clinics, subcutaneous stimulation is deep massage or stimulation using a sophisticated electric vibrator. The machines are generally hand size and have two or more small cylindrical protuberances which vibrate up and down with a frequency and intensity that can be adjusted by the user. They can work wonders where back pain is concerned; but their benefits in treating migraine are less apparent. Some manufacturers of these devices recommend that they be used for a few minutes each day to stimulate the cranial arteries. This is done by placing them on the part of the head most often affected during an attack. Others suggest their use during an attack; for many sufferers, this is impossible. While there is no research we know of to indicate that these devices provide any significant relief for migraine sufferers, neither is there any which shows that they do not. If it works for you, wonderful.

We do, however, have one complaint. An electronics specialist who was asked to examine one of these units informed us that it contained bits and pieces worth perhaps $20.00. Allowing even for labor costs, we calculate that the prices being charged for these machines range from ten to twenty times the cost of production. If, after a discussion with your physician, you consider buying one, do try to arrange a free trial or a money-back guarantee.

SPINAL MANIPULATION

This therapy is engulfed in controversy, whether it is being used by physicians, osteopaths or chiropractors. We know of no research which shows conclusively that it is a routinely useful form of therapy in the treatment of migraine. However, we do know of a number of people who vehemently insist that spinal manipulation "cured" their migraine and should be able to do the same for everyone else. In the absence of any supporting research data, we can only conclude that those who have received total relief from headache were not suffering from migraine in the first place. (Their headaches may have closely mimicked migraine through the referral of pain from the back or neck to the head.) We believe this primarily because it is extremely rare for migraine to be brought on by only one trigger mechanism. Migraine is not *caused* by spinal problems or food sensitivities or anything else: it is an inherited predisposition which exists autonomously within the body and which can be activated into a pain-causing biochemical reaction through the impact of any number of internal or external factors. It is difficult to see how spinal manipulation, however sophisticated, can "cure" migraine which may be triggered by menstruation or by eating chocolate or through variations in barometric pressure. Of course there are exceptions to every rule, and there may well be isolated cases in which migraine was properly diagnosed, and there was only one trigger, and it was capable of removal by spinal manipulation. If that has been your experience, count your blessings. You are a rare and fortunate individual indeed.

There do, however, appear to be a number of cases in which partial relief from true migraine has been realized through this technique. In these cases, a painful back problem amenable to manipulation may have been acting as one of the sufferer's triggers, or a spinal problem may have resulted in an awkward posture which promoted muscle-tension headaches which in turn triggered migraine attacks.

Never subject yourself to any form of manipulation or neck twisting from anyone who does not have professional qualifications. Even those who are professionally trained in the technique must exercise caution because of arteries in the neck which supply blood to the base of the brain; manipulation has on occasion blocked some of these arteries thereby causing a stroke.

Many other forms of supportive therapy for migraine have been suggested in recent years. We have perhaps five hundred of them on file at the Migraine Foundation. They range from the plausible but unproved, such as foot reflexology and Zen, to the implausible and outrageous, including a host of gimmicks such as special poultices, voodoo and tiny pyramids to place under your chair or car seat. Sometimes the expectation of relief through some for of therapy is enough to actually provide some relief—temporarily. But the problem will return unless there is some sound medical basis for the treatment. Still, relief is relief, and we are happy to take it wherever we can find it, always remembering that all-important phrase *"primum non nocere."*

Dr. Arnold Friedman, in one of his talks, put it neatly:

The long-term management of migraine should include: treatment of the whole patient; removal or reduction of precipitating factors; help, where needed, in understanding situational and environmental factors; guidance in resolving any conflicts; the selective and judicious use of medicines and supportive therapies. It is probably through a multiple approach that physicians can offer the migraineur effective therapy.

The patient suffering from the miseries of migraine will try any remedy suggested by physician, friend or fellow-sufferer. There is no single, wholly effective treatment that suits all who suffer; the response to any treatment is highly idiosyncratic, and treatment must, therefore, be carefully tailored to the individual.

CHAPTER 8

Migraine
in
Children

For most adult migraine sufferers, it is a revelation to learn that children share their affliction. This is perhaps because the condition is so often misunderstood; so often linked exclusively to the stresses of living and working, or to complex and very adult neuroses. However, many of these same adults, when asked to think back, will recall experiencing the symptoms during their own childhoods, for migraine often begins at an early age. (One study indicates that 37.5% of patients with classic migraine and 28.5% with common migraine suffered their first attacks before they had reached the age of ten.)

Migraine has been tentatively diagnosed in infants as young as six weeks; but it is much more frequently reported at the ages of two or three years. It is possible, however, that very early migraine is more common than is now understood. Some specialists think it may simply go undiagnosed and unreported because the child has not yet developed the communication skills necessary to describe what he feels.

On the other hand, children do not generally begin eating adult food as a matter of routine until they are at least two years old, and they are thus not exposed to the full range of chemical migraine triggers until then. This, too, could account for a relative absence of reported migraine at earlier ages.

It is known that the pain of migraine attacks in children can be very severe, and there is suspicion that, in some cases, the frightening syndrome in which infants repeatedly bang their heads against walls and the sides of cribs may be related to such pain. What is more certain is that the often miserable behavior of children during the notorious "terrible twos and threes" can, in the case of migrainous children, be attributed in part to their headaches or abdominal pains.

Boys suffer from migraine in greater numbers than girls until the onset of puberty, when the ratio reverses itself as young women begin to experience hormonal changes that can trigger attacks and may begin taking the birth control pill (a potent chemical trigger) either as a means of contraception or as a treatment for acne or other miseries of pubescence. In some cases, young women are not told that the medication they are taking is the contraceptive pill, and this has frequently made correct diagnosis of their headaches more difficult than it might otherwise have been. It should be kept in mind that the changes which accompany puberty are underway within the body some time before the more easily observable physical changes that take place. This, too, can sometimes lead to diagnostic confusion.

Children who experience their first migraine attacks before puberty stand about a fifty-fifty chance of having the problem diminish during adolescence. However it will sometimes return in full force as they enter their twenties.

SYMPTOMS

The symptoms of migraine in children are similar to those experienced by adults, with a couple of significant exceptions. While adults almost invariably turn pale, children may turn red or even become tinged with blue during an attack. Though migraine in adults usually starts on one side of the head, bilateral migraine involving both sides of the head is much more typical in children.

However, symptoms may be quite vague or diffuse, particularly in children from two to five years of age: a nagging irritability; a general feeling of fogginess; withdrawal (sitting quietly in a corner); an absence of normal inquisitiveness and interest in goings on in the immediate surroundings. Children frequently experience migraine pain in the abdomen rather than in the head.

In one study conducted at Toronto's Hospital for Sick Children, 41% of children with migraine experienced associated visual phenomena—the aura of the classic attack. As well as experiencing the blank spots, lights and zigzag lines familiar to adult sufferers, children sometimes perceive themselves as much smaller or much larger than the people around them. They may also experience auditory and visual hallucinations.

If you suspect that your child may be experiencing these visual phenomena, you might wish to provide paper and crayons either during or just after the attack, and ask for a drawing of what was seen. Such drawings could be of assistance to the child's physician or specialist.

Look for: dilated pupils; distended or corded blood vessels on the scalp and on the backs of hands and feet or inside the forearms; swelling of the hands and feet (often difficult to see in chubby toddlers and infants); increased urination; vomiting or nausea; extreme sensitivity to light, sound and strong odors. The child's response to treatment will also provide clues: if he or she has a migraine there will be a favorable response to such comforts as a darkened, quiet room, cold packs, a pillow to raise the head slightly. Often, the child will fall asleep and awaken without the headache. If this doesn't happen, and if the symptoms are severe, you may have a candidate for medication. An understanding physician can help decide.

Stomach pain, car sickness or other motion sickness and nausea and vomiting during periods of intense excitement such as birthdays are also common symptoms among children, even though there may be no related head pain. Often, they forecast the onset of more ordinary migraine symptoms later in life.

Because very young children cannot communicate well, diagnosing their problem is often difficult. Once again, the most important single clue to a proper diagnosis of migraine is family history: if there is a history of recurring headache or migraine anywhere in the child's family, that is the first thing the family physician should know when the child is taken for examination.

TRIGGERS

Children are susceptible to all of the migraine triggers discussed in Chapter 4. While it is true that very young children generally have a carefully restricted diet which limits their exposure to food additives, amines and other triggers, it is also true that those of school age often indulge in chemical-laden junk foods to a much greater extent than adults. Hot dogs (nitrites), hamburgers (MSG), candy and cookies (chocolate) and colas (caffeine and chocolate) are all prime suspects. Watch also for irregular eating time, since migraine attacks can be triggered by low blood sugar.

In very small children still on baby foods, one should suspect anything which "overloads" the senses. Things like very bright light, especially the glare of sunlight reflected off snow or water; strong perfumes or other odors; sharp or loud noises. Wind on the face or head can also trigger migraines. Orange juice or other citrus juices should be suspected, as should any chemical additives that might be found in the infant's food or formula. If the symptoms are very persistent, it may be worth switching to a formula that is not based on cow's milk, such as a soya-based product. The cow's milk could be the problem. Get your physician's approval.

It becomes more difficult to track down migraine triggers in older children, even though their help can be enlisted in the process. (With a little imagination, keeping track can be turned into a kind of game in which even pre-schoolers can get usefully involved.) A few examples from the Migraine Foundation's records will illustrate the kind of detective work that can be involved.

A young schoolgirl suffered a severe headache every Monday, Wednesday and Friday at three o'clock in the afternoon. The school nurse correctly suspected migraine and sought expert advice. In following the girl through one of her headache days, it was discovered that she had the same class each Monday, Wednesday and Friday afternoon, taught by an instructor who habitually wore a heavy, musk-based perfume. The girl's desk was in the front row of the class, close to the perfume-drenched teacher. Moving her desk to the rear of the classroom probably would have solved the problem, but the teacher was understanding and immediately offered to stop wearing the offending scent. The migraines eased. (In general, migrainous children seem to be more sensitive to strong odors than are their adult counterparts.)

Another young girl complained of splitting headaches every day of the week except on the weekends, and always at about two o'clock in the afternoon. In this case, the school nurse had little or no knowledge of migraine and suspected instead that the headaches were in some way psychologically induced. The school psychologist was brought in to try to find the cause. He at first suspected that the girl simply disliked being at school; but she insisted she loved it, and her parents were able to confirm this. Next, the parents became suspect, and the psychologist, in talking with them, suggested that one or the other of them might be harboring attitudes to school that were quite different from the daughter's, thus setting up a subconscious conflict within her that led to the regular headaches. This spawned more than one row between the unfortunate mother and father, as to who was poisoning their daughter's mind. Finally, they sought advice which quickly enabled them to trace the problem to the peanut butter sandwiches the girl insisted on having for lunch every day at school. When the peanut butter was eliminated (over the girl's protests), so were the migraines.

A father who had waited seven years for his son to be old enough to accompany him to baseball games was bitterly disappointed when the boy developed a severe migraine shortly after each game. His mother said it was all the excitement and insisted that the boy stay home. However, a history of migraine in the family led a specialist to suspect that the boy might also be a sufferer. From that point, it did not take long to determine that it was not the excitement of the ball game, but the ritual hot dog that went with it that caused the headaches.

A young skier of some promise often suffered from severe head pain after being on the slopes for a few hours, and this was jeopardizing his chances in the competitions he loved to enter. Migraine was eventually diagnosed, and the prescription was light-polarizing sun glasses which reduced the harsh glare of sunlight reflected off the snow and thereby removed the migraine trigger. Hockey players can have similar problems, particularly if the rink is indoors, where artificial lighting and tobacco smoke can add to the glare problem.

SELECTING A PHYSICIAN

In these and many other cases, parents have been fortunate in having access to expert and understanding advice. Unfortunately, migraine in children is more often than not improperly diagnosed as either something else altogether, or nothing at all—just colic, or growing pains, or fussiness, or a dislike of school, or a sensitive nature or a highly strung personality. In these cases, it is left to the parents or someone else close to the family who knows something about migraine, or perhaps to one of the migraine foundations listed in the back of this book, to provide the initial clue which, ideally, should lead to a consultation with a pediatric neurologist, or a general practitioner with a special interest in migraine. It is, sadly, not unusual for physicians to be unaware that children are susceptible to migraine, and mistaken diagnosis can lead to inappropriate treatment. Parents will need to be careful in selecting a physician.

DRUGS

No one likes to see children taking medication of any sort on a regular basis, and, fortunately, only perhaps a quarter of the children who suffer from migraine require drugs other than an occasional mild analgesic. For some unknown reason, children absorb aspirin into their systems more efficiently than adults, and, frequently, childrens' aspirin will either abort an attack or reduce its severity.

Sometimes, however, more potent medicine is necessary. This is a decision that must be made jointly by the parents and the physician, based on the degree to which the child's migraine attacks are disrupting his or her life. In these cases the initial prescription should be very small (0.3 mg) doses of ergotamine in a combination medication.

ALTERNATIVE THERAPIES

Beyond the ages of three to five years, children react extremely well to training in auto-hypnosis, and to biofeedback and other self-generated techniques of alleviating pain and controlling the vascular system. It hardly needs to be said that such techniques must be tested with extreme caution and only under expert medical supervision. The body's autonomic system is not something to be tinkered with. Nevertheless, such methods may be well worth trying in some cases, particularly where drug therapy may be especially worrisome.

Sleep is often the most effective therapy of all.

NURSING THE CHILD

In addition to the careful administration of such drugs as may be prescribed by a knowledgeable physician, there is much a parent can do to alleviate a migrainous child's suffering.

The first step is, of course, to try to isolate the migraine triggers affecting the child. However, until that can be done—and it cannot always be done with complete success—there will be the problem of treating the headaches when they occur. The child should be put to bed in a quiet, darkened room with a comforting pillow to keep the head slightly elevated. It is important to keep fluid intake up, particularly if vomiting occurs.

Cold packs or compresses applied to the temples and forehead will often ease the pain.

Frequent changing of the cold packs can also be valuable therapy for family members who may be distressed at their helplessness in the face of the youngster's obvious pain.

As soon as the child is old enough to understand, the cause of the pain should be explained to him. Pain from an unknown, unexplained source can be frightening, and children experiencing a severe attack have been known to ask if they are about to die. Others have complained of having a devil in their head. Fear can only complicate their symptoms and make treatment more difficult. A delicate touch is required here: it is obviously important not to make the child think of himself as peculiar or in any way inferior, or to imbue an unhealthy self-pity. Fortunately, this sounds more daunting in prospect than it is in actuality; most parents will find themselves perfectly adequate to the task.

We often hear from parents who are concerned about the psychological problems that can be created in a home where one child has migraine and the others don't, the main fear being that the other children may grow to resent the extra attention given to the migraine sufferer. Here, a straightforward explanation of the nature of migraine should help. Parents must also be careful to avoid making the migrainous child feel guilty should an attack disrupt some family outing or activity.

BEYOND THE HOME

It is also important to explain the child's condition to others with whom he or she has regular contact. Teachers, especially, should know how to recognize an attack. If the child is on medication and is too young to be trusted with the pills, some of the medicine might be left with the school nurse or a reliable teacher if your physician approves. In any case, the proper place for children in the throes of a severe migraine attack is at home, and they should be taken there as soon as possible.

Children who suffer from classic migraine will display symptoms in the pre-headache phase that are difficult to miss once they are understood. They may include impaired reading ability; impaired speech; memory loss and impaired motor abilities. The child may seem "vacant" and inattentive. He or she may be seen shielding the eyes from the light, or blocking out noise with hands over ears. A teacher noticing any of these symptoms can have a quiet word with the child to confirm whether a headache is on its way and then take appropriate action. This may be the administering of the prescribed medication, providing a quiet place to lie down or simply seeing that the child gets home quickly and safely.

Some children who suffer from migraine will be unable to partake in some aspects of the school's physical fitness or sports programs, and this fact must be understood and respected by school authorities. Exercises which involve a head-low position, for example, can sometimes trigger migraine attacks by suddenly increasing the blood flow through the vessels of the scalp.

While an understanding of their child's condition can make it possible for parents to dramatically reduce the frequency and severity of the attacks, parents must also be careful not to over-protect their child. This could lead to isolation from the peer group—condemnation to the bottom of childhood's brutal class structure as someone slightly weird and therefore a legitimate target for harassment and abuse.

Only those who have never had to endure such a sad and lonely childhood experience will argue that it can be in any way constructive.

CHAPTER 9

The Cluster Headache

Cluster headache† differs in several respects from common and classic migraine. These headaches tend to be of relatively short duration—forty-five minutes to two hours long—grouped in series or "clusters" over a period of a few days or weeks, with a subsequent period of freedom from headache which may last a year or more.

Cluster may also appear in the guise of an intense "migraine" of short duration which occurs at precisely the same time, every day, for years on end. This unexplained consistency, with the relative brevity and intensity of the episodes, is what identifies this particular syndrome as cluster rather than migraine.

The pain of cluster can be more severe than all but the worst migraine attacks, giving the condition a reputation as one of the most painful known to medicine. Sufferers frequently report contemplating suicide as a means of escape from the torture, and they sometimes exhibit bizarre or violent behavior during an attack; this may even include self-injury in an attempt to shift the focus of the pain and thus provide a modicum of relief.

†Cluster headache is sometimes called Horton's syndrome or episodic migrainous neuralgia.

Unlike migraine, which occurs more frequently among women than men, cluster headache appears to be an overwhelmingly male affliction, with only about a quarter of the cases reported occurring in women. And cluster is mercifully much more rare than migraine. While migraine is clearly an inherited condition in most instances, there is seldom a family history of cluster headache—though there may be one of migraine. Migraine may begin in early childhood; cluster seldom does; most victims experience their first attacks in their late twenties or early thirties. Cluster attacks tend to strike with baffling regularity at the same time of day (often arousing the victim in the small hours of the morning) and during the same season of the year (although no particular season is favored). They begin suddenly, almost invariably without the warning of the pre-headache symptoms typical of classic or common migraine.

Despite all of these differences, cluster headache is similar to migraine in one important respect—it is a vascular headache in which the pain is related to dilation of the blood vessels of the head. For this reason it is more often than not classified as a sub-species of migraine.

Cluster shares one other significant distinction with migraine: it is far too often improperly diagnosed. Often, by the time a victim receives the correct diagnosis, he has seen a number of doctors and may have had some or all of his teeth extracted by a dentist. His sinuses may have been drained, and he has likely been prescribed eyeglasses. He may have undergone an elaborate and expensive array of uncomfortable and sometimes dangerous testing procedures.

All this, in spite of the fact that cluster headache's symptoms are so typical that the diagnosis can usually be hazarded over the telephone by a knowledgeable physician.

The following graphic account of a cluster attack appeared in a paper by Dr. Lee Kudrow, published in the journal, *Headache:*

Following a period of perhaps several hours during which time I feel quite elated and energetic, I experience a fullness in my ears, somewhat more on the right side than the left, having a character not unlike that which occurs during rapid descent in an airplane or elevator. I next become aware of a dull discomfort, and extension of ear fullness at the base of my skull—further extending over the entire head, on both sides, although somewhat more on the right. At this point, two or three minutes have elapsed; seemingly short, but long enough for me to know that indeed a cluster has begun and will ultimately get worse. Such anticipation causes me considerable consternation regarding any decision to continue my activities or cancel plans and find a place to be alone; giving way to a slowly increasing anxiety, fear, panic and withdrawal. I become aware of myself 'listening' for changes in my head. Is the cluster prematurely aborting itself, progressing further, or unchanging? A sudden stab, only fleeting, strikes my temple, then again—somewhere near the apex of my skull and upper molars in my face—always on the right side. It strikes me again, deep in the skull base and as quickly, changes location to a small area above my eyebrow. My nose is stuffed, yet runs simultaneously. If I could sneeze, I feel the attack would end. But in spite of all tricks I find myself unable to induce sneezing.

While the sharp stabs continue in this fashion, a slow crescendo of dull pain presents itself in an area of a hand's length and breadth over the eye and temporal region. The area of pain narrows into a smaller area but as if magnified, enlarges in intensity. I find myself bending my neck downward, though slightly, as if my head is being gently pushed from behind. My neck up to the base of my skull is tight and feels as if I were wearing a neck collar. I am compelled to remove my tie and loosen my shirt collar even though I know that it will not offer me even a modicum of relief.

In an attempt to alter this persistent discomfort, I drop my head between my legs, while seated. My face and eyes seem to fill with fluid but the pain remains unchanged. In spite of my suntan, as I look into the mirror, a gaunt, sickly pale face peers back. My right eyelid is only slightly drooping, and the white of my eye is charted with many red vessels, giving it an overall colour of pink.

Having difficulty standing in one place too long, I leave

the mirror to continue my alternating pacing and sitting.

As usual, I am struck with the additional fear that the pain will never end, but dismiss it as impossible, since even if it were the case, I would surely die myself.

The pain, now located somewhere behind my eye and slightly above, worsens. The pain is best described as a 'force' pushing with such incredible power through my eye that my head appears to be moving backward, yielding its resistance. The 'force' waxes and wanes, but the duration of successive exacerbations seems to increase. The cluster is at its peak, which is celebrated by an outpouring of tears from my right eye only. I have now been in cluster for thirty-five minutes—ten minutes at its peak.

My wife peeks into the room in which I hold forth. I look up and see her expression of pity, frustration and helplessness. She sees my tortured face as I have seen it in the mirror at this stage before; a drooling mouth, agape, grey face wet on one side, an almost closed eyelid, and smelling of pain and anguish. She closes the door and leaves, feeling hurt for me, anger for the stupidity of medical science and guilt—since deep within her mind is the suspicion that she is the cause of my suffering.

I cry for her, but more for myself. The pain is so incredible. Suddenly I am overwhelmed by a fury. I lift a chair high above my head and crash it to the floor. With a doubled fist I strike the wall. The pain persists.

Waning periods soon become longer in duration and I allow myself to suspect that the peak is behind me—but cautiously, since I have too often been disappointed.

Indeed, the pain is ending. The descent from the mountain of pain is rapid. The 'force' is gone. Only severe pain remains. My nose and eye continue to run. The road back, as with all travel, covers the same territory—but faster. Stabbing, easily tolerated pain is felt. Then gone. Dull, aching fullness, neck stiffness—all disappear in turn, to be replaced by a welcome sensation of pins and needles over the right scalp area—not unlike after one's leg has been 'asleep'. Thus my head has awakened after a nightmare of torment.

Eye and nose dry, I let out a sigh. I collect my pile of wet tissues strewn all over the floor and deposit them in a wastepaper basket. The innocent chair now righted, I rub my bruised fist. Thus, having ended the battle and cleaned up its field, I open the door and enter my pain-free world— until tomorrow.†

We generally recognize three kinds of cluster headache: *periodic, chronic* and *cluster-migraine.* Periodic or episodic is the most common: attacks will occur daily for several weeks and then there will be an extended period of remission. With chronic cluster there is no remission period. Chronic cluster can sometimes evolve out of episodic cluster. The third category is cluster-migraine. This appears to be a transition stage between cluster headache and migraine. In some cases it involves migraine-type headaches having the periodic grouping typical of episodic cluster; in others it is characterized by cluster-type headaches occurring in a migraine-like pattern of single bouts followed by a period of normalcy. However, seasonal common or classic migraine should not be confused with a form of cluster. Migraine can and often does last for days and/or weeks on end, especially in the spring and autumn; but the pain is usually *continuous* in nature which should rule out cluster or migraine-cluster.

The so-called cluster periods, during which attacks occur in episodic-cluster victims, generally last from six to twelve weeks. During this time attacks typically occur one to three times a day, each attack lasting about forty-five minutes. The remission period following a cluster period varies with the individual but averages about twelve months in duration. The pain is confined to one side of the head and is steady, rather than throbbing, as in migraine. Watering of the eye and stuffiness of the nose on the affected side are normal accompaniments. Attacks will often begin on

---

†Lee Kudrow. "Cluster Headache: Diagnosis and Management," *Headache*; April 1979, pp. 142-149. Reprinted by permission of the author.

awakening from an afternoon nap, or an hour or two after falling asleep at night. The behavior of the victim during an attack can provide important clues to diagnosis: pacing, walking, sitting and rocking, shouting or moaning are normal. The typical migraine victim, on the contrary, seeks a dark place in which to lie down and quietly wait out the pain.

The fluctuations in serotonin levels in the blood which seem to play a role in migraine attacks do not occur during cluster headaches. Instead, what has been discovered is a sharp rise in the levels of histamine, which is also a vaso-active amine and can cause blood vessels to swell. This clue, along with the location of the cluster pain behind the eye, the typical shrinking of the pupil and the drooping of the affected eyelid have led to speculation that a release of histamine into the blood causes a swelling of a blood vessel inside the skull known as the internal carotid artery. The walls of this artery carry a network of nerves, which would be compressed as the artery swells, and this would result in pain in the area of the eye. (The portion of the carotid artery in question is known to refer pain to the eye.) Further, among the nerves carried in the wall of this artery are those which control muscle tone in the upper eyelid and the dilation of the pupil of the eye.

Perhaps the most puzzling thing about this condition is that, during a cluster period, almost any substance which is capable of enlarging the blood vessels can cause a headache; but during periods of remission, these same substances have no noticeable effect. Somehow, the sensitivity of the blood vessels involved must be increased during cluster periods.

It has been suggested that this increased sensitivity may be in some way related to previous head injury, which has caused a defect in the nervous system, allowing the blood vessels affected to react with abnormal vigor to histamine and other vaso-active agents. This could explain the predominance of male sufferers, since males are more liable to such injury than females. So far, there is no solid evidence to support this line of speculation.

Alcohol is an effective trigger of cluster headaches, and subjects become extremely sensitive to even small amounts of it during an attack period. And, like migraine, cluster attacks can be brought on by any of a large number of foods and drugs containing substances which can dilate blood vessels. Unlike migraine, stress and emotional upset appear to play only a very minor role in triggering attacks. It is true that some cluster victims suffer from emotional problems to varying degrees; but this is generally a result of the devastating impact of the condition itself. This is particularly true of victims of chronic cluster, who suffer one or more excruciating headaches a day every day for years on end. They are likely to be depressed and demoralized; they may be severely disturbed psychologically. Some will have become addicted to ergotamine and narcotic painkillers which, though ineffective, are still taken every day.

Cluster attacks come and go so suddenly that neither painkillers nor ergotamine taken orally can be fully absorbed by the system in time to provide much relief. By the time these have reached their full potency, the headache is normally receding on its own. Ergotamine taken through an inhaler, in the form of a suppository or by injection is absorbed more quickly and is thus somewhat more effective. But there is a further problem in the treatment of acute attacks, and that is that there may be two or more of these a day, in which case the maximum safe dosage of ergotamine and the more powerful painkillers may be exceeded.

To avoid these problems, many physicians choose to treat cluster headache prophylactically—that is, to prescribe medications which head off attacks before they can occur.

Because of the suspected role of histamine in cluster attacks, some doctors have put their patients on a program of histamine desensitization, in which the sufferer is given daily doses of the substance in order to make his body less sensitive to it during cluster periods. There is now serious doubt as to the effectiveness of this form of treatment. Most specialists now think it does little or no good.

However, there are drugs that do an effective job. Among these, the most widely used in preventing periodic cluster attacks is methysergide. (All of the drugs referred to in this chapter are described in greater detail in Chapter 6.) It provides a clear-cut improvement 70% – 90% of the time.

Lithium carbonate has also been found effective in preventing attacks, particularly in the case of chronic cluster, where it provides a definite improvement in perhaps 85% of cases. Nobody knows why it works. There are side effects, such as lethargy, stomach upset and sometimes a slight trembling in the hands; but most chronic cluster victims are more than happy to put up with these in exchange for relief from their headaches.

Methysergide and lithium carbonate are both powerful drugs and can be used safely only under close medical supervision. But when they are used properly they can make enjoyable once again lives that may have seemed to sufferers scarcely worth continuing. This is especially true where chronic cluster is concerned and where lithium carbonate is the treatment of choice. Neurologist Dr. John Edmeads has noted that: "The need for tight follow-up and the potential risks of lithium deter some physicians from prescribing it. Were these physicians to see the agony of their chronic cluster patients during a headache, and to witness the often dramatic response to lithium, they would use it with alacrity."

Postscript

GUILTY...OR NOT GUILTY

Either consciously or sub-consciously, almost everyone who experiences severe migraine feels *guilty*. Most people don't speak about it as they feel it is something only they experience. Consequently this aspect of migraine is seldom discussed with a physician, and relatively little attention has been paid to this very real problem. Some people create their own guilt, and/or gradually achieve layers of guilt. Some have guilt thrust upon them. Guilt is present almost everywhere:

- the child who feels guilty that in some way he/she is responsible for being at home—for mother having to nurse him, having to quiet brothers and sisters (and unlike the mumps, measles, etc.—it keeps recurring).

- the child who feels guilt returning to school after a day or two absence, who finds it difficult to explain the "illness" to school-mates. (And sometimes to a teacher—one having been known to ask, "What's a strong, healthy girl like you doing with headaches?")

- the teen, who on attending her first formal school dance, vomited over her escort's shoes and tuxedo trousers—and who refused to date for a year or so after (that same boy never did ask her out again).

- the seventeen-year-old who gave concern to her parents because she was bright, attractive, but didn't date or even seem to think about dating—when all the time the girl had such guilt feelings about migraine that she refused dates and eventually discouraged anyone from even asking her.
- the guilt of the young nun who one day was excused from early morning prayers, and was guilty at feeling such relief.
- the guilt of the spouse who could not stand to be with someone who was in pain (and which grew and grew until a divorce resulted). This can extend beyond the family: one gem of a cleaning woman regretfully gave notice as she could not bear to be near anyone in pain.
- the guilt of the man who for ten years insisted that his physician, his family, his co-workers, refer to his "vascular condition" as he refused to say the word "migraine" aloud, for fear of being stigmatized.
- a triangle of guilt—when a father stormed into his son's bedroom and ordered him to get to school or else. The son rose and attempted to dress, but couldn't. The mother was caught between the two, with the father wondering if his son was faking it or not.
- the guilt trip the young bride-to-be was putting on herself as she wondered if it was being fair to marry with her history of migraine.
- the guilt trip a husband experienced who wrote that his wife had had migraines for a year after their marriage, and he wondered if *he* was responsible.
- the deep-seated guilt which occurred with one couple, where one took charge of medication and only doled it out if "it was absolutely needed" . . . the husband looking at his wife as a "jailer" with whom he had to plead to get medication.
- the guilt of the t.v. talk-show host who tried to continue interviewing during a live program. Due to his speech, etc. it was thought he was drunk and his contract was immediately cancelled. Of course the man knew he wasn't drunk, yet felt guilt at having had the migraine attack.

- the guilt of the girl enrolled in an engineering course who was told she had migraines because she was a woman trying to be a man!
- the guilt of the Hollywood actress who had to retire from a promising career because she held up production (and could not get insurance to cover this) when she had a migraine.
- the guilt and fear of the five-year-old boy who heard his mother moaning, "God Take Me Now" one day, and who felt he was somehow responsible.
- the layers upon layers of guilt when a husband raged out of the house one morning leaving behind the ultimatum: "Get rid of that migraine by the time I come home or I am taking the children and leaving you." (Fortunately he did come into the office and talk—and the wife received the help of a neurologist.)
- the guilt and frustration of the woman who periodically had to seek help at the hospital, and whose sister-in-law accused her of being an addict. This resulted in a family feud, some on "one side," some on "the other," and some "wondering."
- the man who tried to hide from his family the fact that he had a migraine attack: his wife felt guilty as she thought he was just being bad-tempered, the children felt guilty not knowing why they were being yelled at to be quiet. The man was finally persuaded to make some sign (hat on backwards, newspaper folded a different way) if he could not come out and voice the problem.
- the mother of the family who allowed herself to be coaxed into going out when she really felt she couldn't. She felt guilt if she "spoiled their fun," and felt guilt if they stayed home because of her. She only felt relief if they went out and left her quietly at home (then the family felt guilty at being out enjoying themselves and not being home looking after mother).
- the woman who, after years of pain, found help from a preventative medication, but who added about 15 pounds—at which point the husband ordered her to give up the "pills or me," as he didn't want a fat slob for a wife.
- a professor who developed migraines on long distance flights, but had convinced himself it was due to guilt at leaving his wife at home. One day he heard a radio program about distance

flights triggering migraines. Now he takes ergotamine before boarding a plane, can handle the migraine and has lost the guilt.

• guilt can involve the neighbors: a migraineur feels guilty about asking that the stereo not be played at top volume. If the neighbors agree one feels one has reduced their sense of enjoyment; if the neighbors do not agree, one feels guilty at the "urge to kill" that accompanies reverberations of extra loud sound.

• guilt occurs when a spouse offers to go anywhere, pay any amount of money, and seek the best help—and yet still the migraines aren't cured. One wonders if one has done everything possible.

• the guilt of a nurse who went into the profession because as a child she had laughed at her mother's "days in bed." She still wonders, now that she also experiences migraines, if she is not being repaid for her lack of understanding as a child.

• one of the largest doses of guilt is measured out to migrainous mothers of young children: the mother wants peace, quiet, rest and yet must tend to her youngsters . . . this type of guilt grows, layer by layer.

• even owners of pets feel guilt: they can't walk the dog that day, the cat must wait for its feeding (did I leave out enough dry food to see it through?).

All of the foregoing, and many, many more case histories are in our files. For every migraineur there is some level of guilt—be it at missing school, a social engagement, disturbing the family, days lost from work, inability to plan vacations or to be present at special events, etc. all of which keep compounding throughout the years.

There are *two* thoughts that go through the mind of *every migraineur* at some time or another:

• why can't I have something like a broken leg that people can see and understand? (Note that sympathy is not asked—just understanding.)

• why can't she/he/they have *five minutes of a migraine, just once* so they'd understand?

MIGRAINE AND THE FAMILY

As is so often the case with migraine, major problems can be handled, but minor ones often escalate out of proportion:
- we can't take mother and father out to a restaurant as he has to be so careful of what he eats, so we only eat at their house and mother never gets away from the stove. He's not being fair to her.

Maybe your mother and father prefer it this way. Or, have you thought of taking her out to lunch separately, or of getting a list of what cannot be eaten and then checking this out with the manager and chef of a proposed restaurant? Or, in good weather, make up a picnic basket based on your mother's suggestions? But, for goodness sake don't let this simmer on the family's emotional burner.

- when migraine is coming on I talk and talk and can't seem to stop. My husband gets so annoyed with me and says I sound as if I'm drunk or on dope.

Over-talkativeness does affect many in the early stages of a migraine. That should/could be a sign to take whatever medication has been prescribed (and/or use whatever therapeutic techniques have been acquired). Get away from everybody, be quiet and rest—talk to the cat, dog or your pillow.

- my physician gives me instructions about what to do at the start of an attack, but what do I do with my two children if I follow these suggestions?

Before the age of the nuclear family, there were often three generations under one roof, so that another adult was available to tend to youngsters. Alternatives must be found.

- see if another family member could be "on call" to help. . .or a close friend who might come and take your children away for an afternoon, etc.
- if attacks are very severe, discuss with your physician, local public health nurse, local area health office, etc. about the possibility of a visiting home-maker (depending on circum-

stances, there may be a fee charged, or insurance/social service agencies may cover all or part of the cost).

• where migraineurs have become acquainted in a community, a form of "buddy" system might be tried, if not arranged through a migraine group, then informally arranged between individuals—with a "you'll take mine today and I'll take yours when you need it" arrangement.

• some communities have a "honorary grandparent" system, whereby lonely elders are linked to lonely children, to their mutual benefit. Perhaps an appeal could be made via a church group, a service club (most of whom welcome new community project ideas) whereby someone would be available.

We've found senior citizens who used to have migraine to be invaluable. Understandably husbands forced to come home from work to see to the children may not be able to do this frequently, and/or may resent it.

• I can manage to feed and look after the basic necessities for my children but how can I make them understand to be quiet, to play outside, etc?

One of the easiest steps we have found is to put *a band-aid* on your forehead; it works equally well for the mother or father in the family, as well as older children, etc. Almost every child from the age of 18 months and up understands a band-aid—it means "hurt," but happily does not imply severe pain, just enough to be understood. Children very quickly pick up the implication and the underlying message that this is a time to play quietly, etc. There is a secondary but equally important reaction to such adhesive bandages; most children have a band-aid put on as a result of a scratch, skinned knees and elbows, etc. Something *inanimate* caused the problem, and a hug or kiss usually accompanied the bandage. We've happily found that when the band-aid is worn, the child does *not* then feel responsible for the pain mother, father, or older sister/brother is feeling.

• I've suffered so all my life, I want to donate my body to science when I die . . . but my family is opposed to this. What can I do?

First check with your family physician who will know what local medical schools, etc. might have provisions for acceptance. Then you'll probably need to check with the school itself, as there are usually certain conditions which must be met (they like as complete a unit as possible). Then once you have the information do talk it over with your minister, priest, rabbi, etc. not only to ascertain religious rules in this regard, but also to help you discuss this, quietly and calmly, with your family, so that if you leave written instructions behind they will be followed. However, it is only honest to point out that such a contribution will almost certainly not be used in regard to migraine specifically, but will serve medicine generally. Meanwhile do check with agencies that serve the blind, kidney disease, etc., as it could well be that specific parts of the body can be used for needed transplants.

• I've had migraine for over twenty years, but last year I experienced a strange sensation in my chest. My family only said, "oh, you've found *another* pain" so I hesitated to go to the doctor. Finally I collapsed and was rushed to hospital for major surgery. Why do one's friends and even family look at you and just see a big "M" for migraine?

This is not that unusual as friends, family (and even on occasion a physician) may be so accustomed to dealing with the migraine that it is easily forgotten that the migraineur is just another person—but one who has recurring headpain. Migraineurs often are their own worst enemy in this regard. They may ignore the first warning signals of something wrong in the body, other than migraine, as over the years they start to "not wanting to bother the doctor." Just because one is migrainous and because for some sufferers, it occupies a part of a life, one must not ignore other symptoms, simply ascribing them to a possible change in character of a migraine, or for fear of being labelled a hypochondriac (when even a nurse's cheery "hello, you here again" can make you want to run from the office.)

During the past forty years, tremendous strides have been taken in the understanding of migraine and in the techniques of treating it. There is still, however, a long way to go before anyone will be able to say that the problem is even under control, let alone solved. How quickly we cover the distance separating us from a complete understanding of the condition and a safe, convenient and reliable means of alleviating its symptoms depends in large measure on how much time and money we wish to devote to the problem. Most researchers involved in the field believe that the long-awaited breakthroughs in understanding migraine are tantalizingly close; a few years of concerted effort, and a focussing of resources, are all that they need.

Much of the research is being undertaken or supported by the many migraine organizations around the world. In the United States the American Association for the Study of Headache publishes a journal appropriately named *Headache,* designed to keep physicians abreast of the latest research. And the National Migraine Foundation's membership is open to both physicians and lay persons: it promotes and finances research projects and provides information to sufferers and their doctors.

In Italy and Scandinavia, physicians with a special interest in migraine have formed organizations to encourage studies and disseminate information.

In Great Britain, there are two excellent organizations: The Migraine Trust—operated by physicians—organizes international symposia and raises funds for research, etc.; the British Migraine Association, founded by a victim of migraine, provides up-to-date information, raises money for research and has also established local branches throughout the United Kingdom.

In the Netherlands, a board composed of physicians, migraine sufferers and interested lay persons has been set up to study how best to serve the needs of sufferers.

In Canada, The Migraine Foundation conducts surveys, encourages research and provides information. It was founded by a migraine sufferer; its board of directors is made up of physicians, people afflicted with migraine and interested lay persons.

In Australia and New Zealand there are, as yet, no national organizations; but there are a number of neurologists attached to hospitals who specialize in the treatment of migraine, and there is reason to hope that a migraine association may be established in the near future.

Partly because of the newness of these groups, partly because of their diversity and partly because of a chronic shortage of money, there is as yet no mechanism through which sufferers in various countries can get together from time to time to discuss their mutual needs and interests. However, it is intriguing to pause and to think for a moment of what the result might be if representatives of a fifth of the world's population were organized into a single body.

In the interval, while awaiting for the answers which must inevitably come, maintaining a sense of humor helps make it all a little more bearable.

I remember the renowned French physician with whom I was chatting at an international conference some time ago, and who startled me by declaring: "In our country we have the answer to migraine. . .the guillotine!"

Nothing can be quite *that* bad. . .

Index